CLINICAL APPROACHES TO TACHYARRHYTHMIAS

edited by

A. John Camm, MD

Volume 18

CLINICAL APPROACHES TO TACHYARRHYTHMIAS

edited by

A. John Camm, MD

St. George's Hospital Medical School
London, United Kingdom

Volume 18

Current Indications for the Implantable Cardioverter Defibrillator

by

Dirk Böcker, MD
Associate Professor of Medicine
University Hospital
Department of Cardiology and Angiology
Münster, Germany

Lars Eckardt, MD
University Hospital
Department of Cardiology and Angiology
Münster, Germany

Günter Breithardt, MD, FESC, FACC
Professor of Medicine and Cardiology
University Hospital
Department of Cardiology and Angiology
Münster, Germany

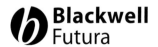
Blackwell
Futura

© 2004 Dirk Böcker, Lars Eckardt and Günter Breithardt
Published by Blackwell Publishing
Blackwell Futura is an imprint of Blackwell Publishing

Blackwell Publishing, Inc., 350 Main Street, Malden, Massachusetts 02148-5020, USA
Blackwell Publishing Ltd, 9600 Garsington Road, Oxford OX4 2DQ, UK
Blackwell Science Asia Pty Ltd, 550 Swanston Street, Carlton, Victoria 3053, Australia

First published 2004

ISBN: 1-4051-27791

Library of Congress Cataloging-in-Publication Data

Böcker, Dirk.
  Current indications for the implantable cardioverter defibrillator / By Dirk Böcker, Lars Eckardt, Günter Breithard.
    p. ; cm. – (Clinical approaches to tachyarrhythmias ; v. 18)
  Includes bibliographical references and index.
  ISBN 1-4051-2779-1 (pbk.)
  1. Cardiovascular instruments, Implanted.   2. Heart–Surgery.
3. Defibrillators.   4. Arrhythmia–Treatment.
  [DNLM: 1. Arrhythmia–therapy.   2. Defibrillators, Implantable. WG 330 C6403 2004 v.18] I. Eckardt, Lars.   II. Breithardt, Günter.   III. Title.   IV. Series.

  RD598.B625 2004
  617.4′120592–dc22
                                                    2004011187
A catalogue record for this title is available from the British Library

Acquisitions: Gina Almond
Production: Katrina Chandler
Set in 11/13 New Century Schoolbook by TechBooks
Printed and bound in India by Replika Press Pvt. Ltd.

For further information on Blackwell Publishing, visit our website:
www.blackwellfutura.com

The publisher's policy is to use permanent paper from mills that operate a sustainable forestry policy, and which has been manufactured from pulp processed using acid-free and elementary chlorine-free practices. Furthermore, the publisher ensures that the text paper and cover board used have met acceptable environmental accreditation standards.

Notice: The indications and dosages of all drugs in this book have been recommended in the medical literature and conform to the practices of the general community. The medications described do not necessarily have specific approval by the Food and Drug Administration for use in the diseases and dosages for which they are recommended. The package insert for each drug should be consulted for use and dosage as approved by the FDA. Because standards for usage change, it is advisable to keep abreast of revised recommendations, particularly those concerning new drugs.

Contents

Introduction

Implantation of defibrillators has evolved dramatically since its introduction by Mirowski in 1980.[1] Technological improvements in devices and leads included a gradual reduction in the size of the device, the introduction of the endocardial approach in 1988, the biphasic waveform and antitachycardia pacing in 1991, pectoral implantation in 1995, inclusion of DDD pacing in 1996 and the delivery of atrial therapies in 1998. Since the first implantation, a huge body of information on the impact of implantable cardioverter defibrillators (ICD) on prognosis has become available, first as observational studies and later as prospective randomized trials. At the present time, we have a large evidence base from the several ICD trials, although it was not always certain that such a large body of ICD evidence would accumulate. Following the MADIT 1 trial[2] in 1996, Fogoros wrote that it should be considered unethical to conduct another ICD trial because "the science does not justify the hazard to participants"[3] (Figure 1).

The objectives of the guidelines are to enhance the appropriateness of practice, improve the quality of cardiovascular care, lead to better patient outcomes, and improve cost effectiveness. The guidelines published by the American Heart Association, the American College of Cardiology, the European Society of Cardiology, and other professional or scientific organizations all have merged evidence from randomized trials and clinical opinion. Especially, in rare diseases such as primary electrical disorders, randomized controlled trials are difficult to conduct and will likely never be done.

The scientific and professional organizations have developed elaborate procedures for the development of consensus guidelines. These include review of clinical trials,

1

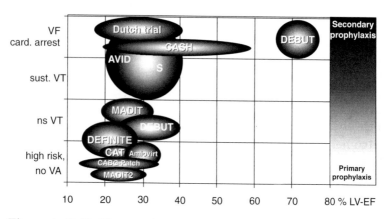

Figure 1. Defibrillator trials.

consideration of clinical practice, consultation and further review, achievement of consensus, announcement of the final document, printing of various national versions of the guidelines, and finally, implementation.[4] However, problems still arise. For example, new important trial results may be published immediately after the guidelines are published. Secondary analyses of clinical trials might yield important information on subgroups. Therefore, evolution of clinical guidelines continues to be a dynamic process. It is influenced by the ongoing publication of trial results and needs frequent updates.

Evolution of Guidelines for Defibrillator Therapy

Guidelines for implantable defibrillators have changed frequently during the last several years. This evolution is due to technological changes in the devices and to several studies that have been published during the last several years. The technological changes that occurred in the 1990s, especially the change from epicardial to transvenous lead systems, the introduction of antitachycardia pacing and biphasic shocks, and the miniaturization of the devices have had a dramatic impact both on the implantation technique and the procedural outcome. Frequent updates in ICD guidelines reflect these technological changes as well as the increasing knowledge on the outcome after ICD implantation in various patient cohorts.

The ACC/AHA pacing guidelines include recommendations on the use of defibrillators since 1991,[5] and have been updated in 1998[6] and 2002.[7] The European guidelines have been around since 1992[8] with the last update having been published in 2001,[9] but newer information is included in the European Guidelines for Prevention of Sudden Cardiac Death, last updated in 2003.[10] These guidelines have been adopted with no or only minor modifications by many national societies and authorities, though at different speeds.[11]

Format of Guidelines

Usually, both American and non-American guidelines use the ACC/AHA classification to express recommendations for indications for device therapy:

- Class I: Conditions for which there is evidence and/or general agreement that a given procedure is useful and effective.
- Class II: Conditions for which there is conflicting evidence and/or a divergence of opinion about the usefulness/efficacy of a procedure or treatment.

- IIa: Weight of evidence/opinion is in favor of usefulness/efficacy.
- IIb: Usefulness/efficacy is less well established by evidence/opinion.
- Class III: Conditions for which there is evidence and/or general agreement that the procedure/treatment is not useful/effective and in some cases may be harmful.

The evidence that supports a recommendation is ranked as level A if the data were derived from multiple randomized clinical trials involving a large number of individuals. The evidence is ranked as level B when the data were derived from a limited number of trials involving a smaller number of patients or from well-designed data analyses of nonrandomized studies. Evidence from observational data registries is ranked as level B in the ACC/AHA classification[12] and only as level C in the ESC guidelines.[9] Evidence is ranked as level C when the consensus opinion of experts was the primary source of recommendation. This does not necessarily mean that a recommendation, which is based on level C evidence, is worse than one based on level A evidence. Especially in patient cohorts with rare diseases, such as long QT syndrome or hypertrophic obstructive cardiomyopathy (HOCM), randomized trials will be difficult to conduct and possibly never be done.

Background of ICD therapy

Aims of ICD Therapy

The primary aim of ICD therapy is prevention of sudden cardiac death, which in the majority of cases is due to ventricular tachyarrhythmias.[13,14] The ICD is able to detect and terminate the arrhythmia by antitachycardia pacing or electric shock delivery and to pace in case of bradycardia. There are secondary aims of ICD therapy. In cases of stable and hemodynamically tolerated ventricular tachycardia, arrhythmia may be terminated by antitachycardia pacing, which can occur without patient awareness of the arrhythmia. Expectation of reliability of the ICD in the protection against sudden cardiac death may contribute to the quality of life of the patient and his environment.

Clinical Efficacy of ICD Therapy

Implantable defibrillators were originally developed for the prevention of sudden cardiac death in patients with frequent ventricular fibrillation or symptomatic ventricular tachycardia.[1] Efficacy has been estimated by the termination of symptomatic ventricular tachyarrhythmias assuming that the majority of those would have been fatal without immediate termination by the devices.[15–18] These early studies, which used defibrillator discharges as surrogate mortality events, tended to overestimate the benefit from device implantation. When devices with extended memory functions became available, device discharges could be replaced by proven ventricular tachyarrhythmias above a certain rate.[19,20] All these studies suggested a very high efficacy of defibrillator implantation for secondary prevention of sudden cardiac death. It has also been suggested early on that the benefit from ICD implantation might be greater in patients with a more advanced cardiac disorder rather than in patients with a more preserved left ventricular function.[21] However, there has been a controversy in this discussion.[22] These observational studies have now been supplemented with large randomized trials comparing the efficacy of ICD implantation to beta-blocker therapy[23] and/or to amiodarone therapy[23–25] in survivors of sudden cardiac death or patients with symptomatic ventricular tachycardias in the presence of severely depressed left ventricular function. Device discharges or documented ventricular tachyarrhythmias as surrogates for mortality events now have increasing importance in studies trying to show the efficacy of drug therapy[26] or ablation therapy under the safety net of an implanted device.

Alternatives to ICD Therapy

Pharmacologic alternatives to ICD therapy include class I, II, and III antiarrhythmic agents. Beta-adrenergic blockers reduce mortality and sudden death in patients convalescing from myocardial infarction and in patients with heart failure. Their role in suppression of recurrences of ventricular tachyarrhythmias in secondary prevention is less clear.[27] The notion that class I antiarrhythmic drugs might save lives by suppressing the triggers of life-threatening ventricular arrhythmias was proven incorrect when the Cardiac Arrhythmia Suppression Trial (CAST) demonstrated that patients whose ventricular ectopics were successfully suppressed by a number of class I antiarrhythmic drugs died more readily than similar patients who were treated with placebo.[28,29] Attention then shifted to class III agents. However, the class I agent, quinidine, continues to be advocated for the treatment of patients with idiopathic ventricular fibrillation by a group from Israel.[30]

Amiodarone and sotalol have been shown to be superior to class I agents. In the post-myocardial infarction patients, empiric amiodarone has been shown to reduce arrhythmic mortality but the benefit with respect to total mortality in such patients with left ventricular dysfunction is less clear.[31,32] There is some evidence from secondary analyses of amiodarone trials that a combination therapy of amiodarone and beta-blockers is more effective than amiodarone alone.[33] However, this hypothesis has never been tested in a larger prospective randomized trial.

Long-term treatment with antiarrhythmic drugs continues to be problematic; especially amiodarone, which is frequently discontinued because of adverse effects.

Catheter ablation has most often been used as an adjunctive therapy in patients with frequent episodes of ventricular tachycardia[34] and even in some patients with frequent episodes of ventricular fibrillation.[35] New mapping systems and improved ablation strategies allow for mapping and ablation of tachyarrhythmias even if these are not well tolerated.[36] With continuing improvement of ablation technology and changes in ablation strategies, it might be conceivable that ablation therapy could not only complement defibrillator therapy but even replace it at least in subsets of patients. Currently, the highest efficacy rates are still in idiopathic left ventricular tachycardia, bundle brunch reentrant tachycardia, and in right ventricular outflow tract tachycardia, in all of which ablation is preferable to ICD therapy.[37]

Comparison of Drugs and Devices

Direct comparison of antiarrhythmic drugs and device therapy has been performed in several retrospective nonrandomized reports. ICD therapy has been shown to be superior both to electrophysiologically guided sotalol[38] as well as empiric amiodarone.[39] More recently, a series of prospective studies, which compared antiarrhythmic drug therapy to implantation of ICDs, has been published. The most important comparison is that of amiodarone versus defibrillators. This comparison was done in AVID,[25] CASH,[23] CIDS[24] and AMIOVIRT.[40] Some other trials compared ICD therapy to "conventional" therapy,[2] which consisted of a variety of antiarrhythmic drugs or even including other antiarrhythmic interventions such as VT surgery[41] making it much more difficult to draw firm conclusions. And finally, a few trials compared ICD therapy to no antiarrhythmic therapy[2,42,43] or only beta-blocker therapy,[24,44] coming as close as possible to a placebo arm.

Studies that compared ICD to amiodarone therapy in patients with aborted sudden death or symptomatic ventricular tachycardia and the MADIT study have demonstrated the lifesaving efficacy of ICD therapy and its superiority compared to conventional medical management in treating patients at high risk of sudden arrhythmic death. These trials have put an end to the discussion whether ICDs can reduce mortality or merely change the mode of death from arrhythmic death to death from progressive heart failure.

The trials have highlighted two important concepts related to the efficacy of ICD therapy: (1) Patients with advanced LV dysfunction benefit to a greater extent than patients with a better preserved LV systolic function. This is probably because patients with a greater LV systolic impairment have higher absolute rates of death, thus receiving more evident absolute benefit. (2) Only patients who have a high arrhythmic death rather than a high non-arrhythmic death rate can derive a benefit from ICD implantation. Currently, our ability to terminate ventricular fibrillation or ventricular tachycardia and thus prevent sudden cardiac death is now much superior to our risk stratification strategy and our ability to identify the individual patient who is truly at high risk of ventricular tachyarrhythmias.[45] These trials have produced varying results that have largely depended on the underlying cardiac disease and the presenting arrhythmia as well as additional inclusion criteria that were used for risk stratification. Therefore, the results of ICD therapy, which form the basis for therapeutic decisions, will be presented separately for each underlying disease.

Current Indications for ICD Therapy

Contraindications to ICD Therapy

ICD therapy is not appropriate in cases where the cause of the arrhythmia is transient or reversible, e.g., during an evolving acute myocardial infarction. Curative therapy should always be considered first, followed by defibrillator implantation with its potential drawbacks. Catheter ablation in a patient with WPW syndrome is a good example, as well as surgical ablation in well-selected patients with an old infarction with relatively preserved left ventricular function, a well-circumscribed aneurysm, and inducible monomorphic ventricular tachycardia. Patients with acute ischemia are preferably treated with revascularization (Figure 2).

In general, patients with a short life expectancy, arbitrarily of 6 months or less, are not appropriate candidates for ICD implantation. Psychiatric disorders may seriously interfere with the acceptance of ICD therapy and with ICD follow-up in the outpatient clinic.

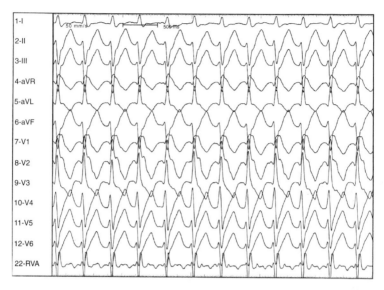

Figure 2. Typical idiopathic left ventricular tachycardia with RRB, inferior axis configuration that was successfully ablated at the left posterior fascicle.

ICD Therapy in Specific Disease States

The underlying disease has a major impact on patient prognosis. It will influence the decision to implant an ICD earlier or later in the treatment algorithm. Therefore, the results of ICD therapy will be discussed in relation to the underlying cardiac disease.

CAD

Patients with coronary artery disease, many of them survivors of acute myocardial infarction, represent the majority of patients at risk of sudden cardiac death in most clinical practices. These patients have an increased risk of developing malignant ventricular tachyarrhythmia. In some of them, the risk is high enough to justify the implantation of a defibrillator. Therefore, risk stratification of this patient group is of major importance.

Risk stratification

LV function. Reduced left ventricular ejection fraction continues to be the most important single factor for risk stratification after myocardial infarction. It has formed the basis for risk stratification in several trials of ICD implantation either together with arrhythmia markers (late potentials in the signal-averaged ECG[46] or nonsustained ventricular tachycardias,[2,47] with markers of autonomic dysfunction,[48] or alone.[42]

Signal-averaged ECG. Abnormalities in the signal-averaged ECG have traditionally been used as a marker for an increased risk for the occurrence of ventricular tachycardias, not so much to indicate an increased risk for ventricular fibrillation.[49–51] In addition to a reduced LV function, they were used to select patients for the CABG Patch trial. The CABG Patch trial compared prophylactic implantation of a cardioverter defibrillator (ICD) implantation with no antiarrhythmic therapy in patients undergoing coronary bypass surgery who had a left ventricular ejection fraction <0.36 and an abnormal signal-averaged ECG.[46] Nine hundred patients were intraoperatively randomly assigned to therapy with an implantable cardioverter defibrillator (446 patients) or to the control group (454 patients). The primary endpoint of the study was overall mortality. There were 102 deaths among the 446 ICD group patients and 96 deaths among the 454 control group patients, a hazard ratio of 1.07 ($P = 0.63$). ICD therapy reduced arrhythmic death by 45%.

However, cumulative arrhythmic mortality at 42 months was only 6.9% in the control group and only 4.0% in the ICD group ($P = 0.057$). Because 71% of the deaths were non-arrhythmic, total mortality was not significantly reduced.[52]

Heart rate variability. Heart rate variability (HRV) is considered as a noninvasive tool to assess cardiac autonomic tone at the level of the sinus node. Numerous estimates for HRV have been proposed and investigated since the landmark study in 808 infarct survivors by Kleiger et al.[53] They showed that patients with a severely impaired heart rate variability (defined as a 24-hour standard deviation of the NN intervals [SDNN]) <50 ms had the worst prognosis compared to an intermediate risk group (SDNN 50–100 ms) and a low-risk group (SDNN > 100 ms). The first prospective evaluation of heart rate variability (together with baroreflex sensitivity) was done in the ATRAMI trial (Autonomic Tone and Reflexes After Myocardial Infarction),[54] which enrolled 1284 patients with a recent (<28 days) myocardial infarction. Subsequently, reduced heart rate variability was implemented in an interventional trial with prophylactic ICD implantation in patients with a recent myocardial infarction. This Defibrillator In Acute Myocardial Infarction Trial (DINAMIT)[48] aimed to enroll patients shortly after their infarction (day 6 to day 40) who have reduced left ventricular function (LVEF ≤ 0.35) and impairment of cardiac autonomic function shown by depressed heart rate variability (SDNN ≤ 70 ms) or elevated average 24-hour heart rate (mean 24-hour R-R interval ≤ 750 ms, assessed by Holter monitoring). Six hundred and seventy-four patients with a mean ejection fraction of 28% and a peak CK level of approximately 2300 U/l were then randomized to receive an ICD in addition to the best medical therapy or the best medical therapy alone including aspirin, beta-blockers, ACE inhibitors, and statins. The trial's endpoint was total mortality. Patients treated with an ICD had a 58% lower arrhythmic mortality that was counterbalanced by an increase in nonarrhythmic mortality of 75%. Total mortality (6.9% per year in the control group) was not changed by prophylactic ICD implantation.[55]

Baroreflex sensitivity. Baroreflex sensitivity (BRS) using the phenylephrine method was introduced as a clinical method of assessing vagal reflex activity. Together with heart rate variability, BRS was prospectively evaluated in the ATRAMI trial.[54] This multicenter international prospective study enrolled 1284 patients with a recent (<28 days) myocardial infarction who were followed for 21 (SD 8) months. The primary endpoint was cardiac mortality. Low values of either heart rate variability (SDNN < 70 ms) or BRS (<3.0 ms per mmHg) carried a significant multivariate risk of cardiac mortality (3.2 and 2.8, respectively). The association of low SDNN and BRS increased the risk further; the 2-year mortality was 17% when both were below the cut-offs and 2% ($P < 0.0001$) when both were well preserved (SDNN > 105 ms, BRS > 6.1 ms per mmHg). The association of low SDNN or BRS with LVEF below 35% carried a relative risk of 6.7 (3.1–14.6) or 8.7 (4.3–17.6). These findings suggest that impaired BRS and reduced HRV are not merely exchangeable risk stratifiers but rather are additive prognostic indices in patients after myocardial infarction, especially in those patients with a reduced LV function.

Baroreflex sensitivity has never been used as a risk stratifier in a defibrillator trial.

Heart rate turbulence. Heart rate turbulence (HRT), representing fluctuations of the sinus rhythm cycle length after a single ventricular premature beat, has recently been introduced as a new autonomic risk marker. The fluctuations are characterized by two numerical parameters, termed turbulence onset and turbulence slope. Heart rate turbulence is critically vagal dependent and highly correlated with spontaneous baroreflex sensitivity.[56–58] The method was validated using the population of the Multicentre Post-Infarction Program (MPIP) and the placebo population of the European Myocardial Infarction Amiodarone Trial (EMIAT).[59] The validation study revealed as optimal dichotomy points 0% for HRT onset and 2.5 ms/RR interval for heart rate turbulence slope. Subsequent data analyses of ATRAMI[60] confirmed that combining heart rate turbulence, baroreflex sensitivity, and heart rate variability (SDNN), in a composite autonomic index was the strongest predictor. The relative risk was 16.79 if all four factors were abnormal. In a multivariate analysis, however, only abnormal turbulence onset and turbulence slope, and left ventricular ejection fraction remained as independent predictors. More recently, heart rate turbulence was prospectively validated in a cohort of 1455 survivors of acute myocardial infarction who were in sinus rhythm.[61] Patients were classified into the following HRT categories: category 0 if both turbulence onset and turbulence slope were normal, category 1 if either turbulence onset or turbulence slope was abnormal, or category 2 if both turbulence onset and turbulence slope were abnormal. The primary endpoint was all-cause mortality. Multivariately, heart rate turbulence category 2 was the strongest predictor of death (hazard ratio, 5.9), followed by LVEF $\leq$ 30% (hazard ratio, 4.5), diabetes mellitus (hazard ratio, 2.5), age $\geq$65 years (hazard ratio, 2.4), and heart rate turbulence category 1 (hazard ratio, 2.4).

Like baroreflex sensitivity, heart rate turbulence has not been used as a criterion for risk stratification in a trial of ICD implantation.

Microvolt level T-wave alternans. Microvolt-TWA assesses subtle changes in ventricular repolarization, a heart-rate-dependent increase in spatial dispersion of repolarization. It has been shown to correlate closely to arrhythmia induction in the electrophysiology laboratory. In the first prospective study in 95 ICD recipients,[62] TWA was compared with invasive EP testing, LVEF, baroreflex sensitivity, signal-averaged ECG, analysis of 24-hour Holter monitoring, and QT dispersion from the 12-lead surface ECG with respect to their ability to predict the recurrence of ventricular tachyarrhythmia as documented by ICD electrograms. In a multivariate analysis, TWA was the only statistically significant independent risk factor.

The usefulness of microvolt TWA for risk stratification in survivors of acute myocardial infarctions is controversial. In a study by Tapanainen et al.[63] in 379 consecutive patients, TWA as well as other noninvasive risk predictors were measured. Sustained TWA was found in 56 patients (14.7%), none of whom died. In a multivariate analysis, the incomplete TWA test (inability to perform exercise or inability to reach a heart rate >105 bpm) was the most significant predictor of cardiac death (relative risk 11.1). They concluded that sustained TWA during the predischarge exercise test after AMI did not indicate an increased mortality risk.

In contrast, Ikeda et al. studied 102 patients who were able to complete the tests. The combined assessment of TWA and late potentials was associated with a high positive predictive value for an arrhythmic event after acute myocardial infarction whereas for TWA alone, its sensitivity and negative predictive value in predicting arrhythmic events were very high.[64]

Like baroreceptor reflex sensitivity and heart rate turbulence, TWA measurements have not been used for risk stratification in an intervention study (e.g., ICD trial).

Secondary prevention of cardiac arrest or sustained ventricular tachycardias in patients with coronary artery disease

Four prospective randomized trials have exclusively or predominantly included patients with coronary artery disease. The first of these studies and the first defibrillator study to be done in secondary prevention after aborted sudden death was the Dutch cost-effectiveness study.[41] This study tested the effectiveness of ICD implantation as first-choice therapy versus the conventional electrophysiology-guided therapeutic strategy of starting with antiarrhythmic drugs and using the ICD only as a last resort. Sixty consecutive survivors of cardiac arrest after myocardial infarction were assigned to both treatment arms and were followed for a median of 24 months. Primary endpoints (main outcome events, including death, recurrent cardiac arrest, and cardiac transplantation), number of invasive procedures and antiarrhythmic therapy changes, and duration of hospitalization were compared. In the early ICD group, four patients (14%) died, all from cardiac causes. The total number of deaths in the conventional group was 11 patients (35%): four died suddenly, five died of heart failure, and two died of non-cardiac causes. In addition, 16 conventionally treated patients underwent late ICD implantation. These data suggest that ICD implantation as first choice would be preferable to the conventional approach in survivors of cardiac arrest caused by old myocardial infarction. It should be mentioned that the conventional therapeutic strategy included class I drugs, sotalol, or VT surgery in a few patients each. The strategy of ICD implantation as first-choice therapy was also more cost effective.[65] The investigators calculated a net cost-effectiveness of $11,315 per patient per year alive saved by early ICD implantation. Costs in the early ICD group were higher only during the first 3 months of follow-up, but as a result of the high proportion of therapy changes, including arrhythmia surgery and late ICD implantation, costs in the EP-guided strategy group became higher after that. Invasive therapies and hospitalization were the major contributors to costs. If quality-of-life measures are taken into account, the cost-effectiveness of early ICD implantation was even more favorable.

Following this trial, three other trials, which share many similarities, have been published. These are the Antiarrhythmics Versus Implantable Defibrillators study (AVID),[25] the Canadian Implantable Defibrillator Study (CIDS),[24] and the Cardiac Arrest Study Hamburg (CASH).[23]

AVID was the largest of these studies. It included 1016 patients with resuscitated ventricular fibrillation (45%) or sustained ventricular tachycardia (55%). Patients with ventricular tachycardia also had either syncope or other serious cardiac symptoms, along with a left ventricular ejection fraction ≤40%. Eighty-one percent of these patients had coronary artery disease. The patients were randomly assigned to treatment with class III antiarrhythmic drugs (in all but 74 empiric amiodarone) or implantation of a cardioverter defibrillator. The primary endpoint was overall mortality.

Overall survival was greater with the implantable defibrillator, with unadjusted estimates of 89.3%, as compared with 82.3% in the antiarrhythmic drug group at 1 year, 81.6% versus 74.7% at 2 years, and 75.4% versus 64.1% at 3 years ($P < 0.02$). The corresponding reductions in mortality with ICD were 39 ± 20%, 27 ± 21%, and 31 ± 21%. The results of AVID were consistent among all prespecified subgroups: CAD versus other diseases, VF versus VT, all age groups, and all ejection fractions. However, there was a small trend toward a lesser benefit in patients with an ejection fraction above 35%. The Canadian Implantable Defibrillator Study (CIDS)[24] had very similar inclusion and exclusion criteria. Predominantly, patients after resuscitated VF or symptomatic VT were included, but in contrast to AVID and CASH, patients with unmonitored syncope and inducible ventricular tachycardia were also included into the trial. A total of 659 patients were randomly assigned to treatment with the ICD or with amiodarone, far more than the initially planned 400 patients.[66] The primary outcome measure was all-cause mortality, and the secondary outcome was arrhythmic death. At 5 years, 85.4% of patients assigned to amiodarone were still receiving it at a mean dose of 255 mg/day. However, there was a significant crossover rate. Of the ICD patients 28.1% were also receiving amiodarone, and 21.4% of amiodarone patients had received an ICD. In CIDS, the reduction in mortality did not reach statistical significance. A non-significant reduction in the risk of death was observed with the ICD, from 10.2% per year to 8.3% per year (19.7% relative risk reduction; $P = 0.142$) and a non-significant reduction in the risk of arrhythmic death was observed, from 4.5% per year to 3.0% per year (32.8% relative risk reduction; $P = 0.094$). The third study, which was run at the same time and included a similar type of patients, was the Cardiac Arrest Study Hamburg, CASH.[23] CASH differed from AVID and CIDS in two respects: it had a beta-blocker arm, which was as close as possible to a true placebo arm, and it initially also had a second drug arm utilizing propafenone. CASH was the first of these studies to start and the last to finish. Only survivors of cardiac arrest resulting from documented ventricular tachyarrhythmias were included. After inclusion of 230 patients that were randomly assigned to propafenone, amiodarone, metoprolol, or the implantable defibrillator, the propafenone arm of CASH was stopped because of excess mortality compared with the implantable defibrillator group.[67] A significantly higher incidence of total mortality, sudden death (12%), and cardiac arrest recurrence or sudden death (23%) was found in the propafenone group (based on intention-to-treat) compared with the implantable defibrillator-treated patients (0%, $P < 0.05$).

The study was continued with three arms until 1998 when 288 patients in the three remaining arms were included and were followed for a minimum of 2 years. Over a mean follow-up of 57 ± 34 months, the crude death rates were 36.4% in the ICD and 44.4% in the combined amiodarone/metoprolol arm. Overall survival was higher, though not significantly, in patients assigned to ICD than in those assigned to drug therapy ($P = 0.081$, hazard ratio 0.766). In ICD patients, the percentage of reductions in all-cause mortality were 41.9%, 28.4%, 22.8% at years 1, 3, and 5, respectively. Data from AVID, CIDS and CASH (only amiodarone and ICD arms) were merged into a meta-analysis.[68] This analysis showed a significant reduction in death from any cause with the ICD with a summary hazard ratio of 0.72. This 28% reduction in the relative risk of death with the ICD was almost entirely due to a 50% reduction in arrhythmic death. Survival was extended by a mean of 4.4 months by the ICD over a follow-up period of 6 years. Patients with left ventricular ejection fraction ≤35% derived significantly more benefit from ICD therapy than those with better preserved left ventricular function.

This was also found in a post hoc analysis of CIDS.[69] This analysis showed that three clinical risk factors, age ≥70 years, left ventricular ejection fraction ≤35%, and New York Heart Association class III or IV, predicted the risk of death and benefit from the ICD. Quartiles of risk were constructed, and the mortality reduction associated with ICD treatment in each quartile was assessed. In the highest risk quartile, there was a 50% relative risk reduction of death in the ICD group, whereas in the three lower quartiles, there was no benefit. Patients who are most likely to benefit from an ICD could be identified with a simple risk score (≥2 risk factors). Thirteen of 15 deaths that were prevented by the ICD occurred in patients with ≥2 risk factors. The cost per life-year gained in patients with ≥2 factors was C$ 65,195, compared with C$ 916,659 with <2 risk factors.[70]

Following these trials, episodes of ventricular fibrillation or symptomatic ventricular tachycardias in patients with poor left ventricular function have been classified as a class I indication for ICD implantation (Figure 3).

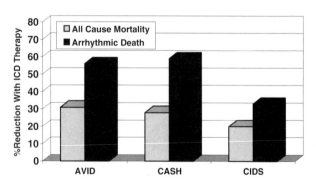

Figure 3. Relative risk reduction in secondary prevention trials.

It should be mentioned though, that patients with a history of hemodynamically tolerated ventricular tachycardias were not included in any of these trials, nor is a prospective trial for these patients available. For these patient cohorts only observational data or data from registries are available. In a small study, we showed that patients who initially presented with a stable VT without syncope had much faster (>240/min and more than 50 ms faster than the initial tachycardia) VTs during follow-up.[20] In the AVID registry, which included all patients who could not be entered into the study, there was no difference in outcome between patients who were asymptomatic at their initial presentation and those who had presented with VF,[71] confirming in some other way our previous results. However, also in the registry, patients with a preserved LV ejection fraction of >35% had a better prognosis with a relatively low event rate.

Primary prevention of sudden cardiac death after myocardial infarction

The indications for implantation of an ICD for primary prevention after myocardial infarction are based on three major studies. Two of them, Multicenter Automatic Defibrillator Implantation Trial (MADIT)[2] and MADIT II,[42] were designed to investigate the effect of prophylactic ICD implantation while the third, MUSTT,[47] was designed to investigate the effect of an EP-guided therapeutic strategy.

The Multicenter Automatic Defibrillator Implantation Trial II (MADIT II)[42] was designed to investigate whether the ICD would be effective in the prevention of all-cause death in patients after myocardial infarction with a low ejection fraction (≤30%). The study was based on the assumption that ICD would reduce all-cause deaths by 38% at 2 years with a 95% power and a

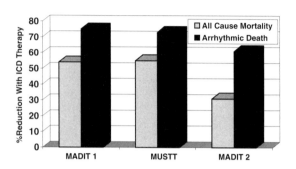

Figure 4. Relative risk reduction in primary prevention trials.

probability value of 0.05. A randomization ratio of 3:2 to receive an ICD or conventional therapy was selected. Analysis of the primary endpoint was performed using a triangular sequential design, similar to the one adopted in the MADIT trial.

After inclusion of 1232 patients, MADIT II was terminated because of a significant (31%) reduction in all-cause death in patients assigned to ICD therapy. MADIT II provides evidence that patients meeting the entry criteria have a better survival if they receive a prophylactic ICD (Figure 4).

After publication of MADIT II, the Food and Drug Administration approved the use of a Guidant ICD for this indication. Many professional organizations[7,10,11] updated their guidelines recommending the trial's inclusion and exclusion criteria as a class IIa in dication for prophylactic ICD implantation. However, concern was also raised because less selective implantation criteria could result in many patients receiving ICDs who did not stand to benefit from the implantation, exposing some patients to unnecessary risks and using societal resources less efficiently.[72] There are different estimates for the increase in implantation rates according to the MADIT II selection

Table 1. *Clinical characteristics and observed efficacy in published trials.*

	Follow-up (months)	NYHA I	NYHA II	ACE-I	Beta-blocker	Absolte RR
MADIT	27	33%	50%	60%	25%	23.4%
MADIT II	20	35%	35%	70%	70%	5.6%
AVID	18	50%	43%	68%	29%	6.9%
CIDS	24	60%	30%	70%	27%	4.3%

criteria. From the German PreSCD registry, a registry of more than 5000 myocardial infarction survivors in cardiology practice outside hospitals, it was estimated that about 5% of all survivors of myocardial infarction have an ejection fraction of $\leq 30\%$, thus fulfilling the MADIT II selection criteria. These criteria include five times more patients than the MADIT/MUSTT criteria, which require arrhythmia and inducibility in addition to a low ejection fraction. Plummer et al. estimated that application of the MADIT II selection criteria would increase the number of patients fulfilling national implantation criteria from about 150/million to 504/million ("new incidence") and 311/million ("prevalence") per year,[73] which is in excess of the current implantations in Britain by a factor of almost 20 (see Table 1).

Both from MADIT and MADIT II, it is known that those patients with the most advanced left ventricular dysfunction benefit more than those with a better cardiac function. In a post hoc analysis, Moss et al. found that patients with an ejection fraction of less than 26% had far greater benefit from ICD implantation than patients with an ejection fraction between 26% and 35%.[74] Later they identified three independent risk factors: ejection fraction <26%, QRS duration $\geq$120 ms, and a history of heart failure treatment.[75] The benefit from ICD treatment increased with the number of risk predictors. Patients at the highest mortality risk (all three risk factors; hazard ratio 4.33) achieved the largest mortality reduction (hazard ratio 0.20) from defibrillator therapy. Thus, in patients with chronic coronary heart disease, the magnitude of the survival benefit from the implanted defibrillator is directly related to the severity of cardiac dysfunction and its associated mortality risk. The same was found in a post hoc analysis of the MUSTT patients.[76] In this analysis, a filtered QRS duration >114 ms in the signal-averaged ECG identified patients at higher risk of arrhythmic death or cardiac arrest. The combination of an ejection fraction ≤30% and an abnormal signal-averaged ECG identified a subgroup of particularly high risk, consisting of 21% of the total study population. And finally, also in MADIT II, it was found that those patients with a wider QRS complex had a higher benefit from ICD implantation.[77] A 49% reduction in mortality was found in one-half of MADIT II patients with QRS ≥ 120 ms (HR = 0.51; $P = 0.07$). In the one-third of MADIT II patients who had a QRS > 120 ms, the reduction was even higher, 63% ($P = 0.004$). This observation was reinforced by a significant association between QRS duration considered as a continuous variable with benefit of ICD. It is worth emphasizing that in patients with QRS < 120 ms, there was still a substantial reduction in mortality (29%) with ICD therapy.

In contrast to MADIT and MADIT II where 85% of the patients were >6 months post myocardial infarction, DINAMIT, which included patients within the first month after a myocardial infarction failed to demonstrate the benefit from prophylactic ICD implantation despite the fact that most patients had a large anterior infarct with a rather depressed left ventricular ejection fraction of 28%

mean. The 58% reduction in arrhythmic death was coun-terbalanced by a 75% increase in nonarrhythmic deaths.[55] However, the results of MADIT II were confirmed by the Sudden Cardiac Death in Heart Failure Trial (SCD-HeFT),[78] which did show a significant 23% reduction in total mortality in chronic heart failure patients regard-less of the underlying etiology (for further details see below).

DCM

Secondary prevention of cardiac arrest or sustained ventricular tachycardias in nonischemic dilated cardiomyopathy
In contrast to patients with coronary artery disease, risk stratification in patients with idiopathic dilated cardio-myopathy is much more difficult. In addition, these pa-tients are underrepresented in the ICD studies of sec-ondary prevention. In AVID, CASH, and CIDS only 15%, 11%, and 10%, respectively, of all patients had idiopathic dilated cardiomyopathy. All these studies showed a reduc-tion of total mortality in patients with nonischemic dila-ted cardiomyopathy of 20–40% compared to conven-tional therapy.[23–25] However, the confidence interval for patients with nonischemic dilated cardiomyopathy was much longer than for patients with coronary artery disease.

In the meta-analysis that combined the results of these three studies, only 225 of 1832 patients had nonis-chemic cardiomyopathy.[68] These patients showed a haz-ard ratio for the reduction of total mortality of 0.78, which was very similar to the total cohort (0.72). How-ever, the 95% confidence interval for these patients ranged from 0.45 to 1.37. It should also be mentioned that only between 0% and 23% of the amiodarone-treated patients and between 0% and 53% of the ICD-treated patients also received a beta-blocker at discharge. Nevertheless, ICD implantation for secondary prevention after aborted sudden cardiac death, with documented ventricular fibrillation or with sustained ventricular tachycardias, is well accepted. The significance of syncope without documented ventricular arrhythmias is still unclear. A nonrandomized study showed similar event rates of appropriate ICD discharges in patients who received an ICD because of syncope and patients who received a defibrillator after aborted sudden death or episodes of ventricular tachycardia or fibrillation.[79] Another study showed significantly lower event rates in a series of consecutive patients treated with an ICD compared to conventionally treated patients.[80] It, therefore, seems reasonable to treat patients with nonischemic dilated cardiomyopathy and syncope similar to those after aborted sudden cardiac death if other causes of syncope are excluded.

Primary prevention of sudden cardiac death
Total mortality increases with progressive left ventricular dysfunction. Also, the number of sudden cardiac deaths increases with progressive left ventricular dysfunction. However, the proportion of nonsudden deaths, especially death from progressive heart failure, increases even more. Obviously, in patients with nonischemic dilated cardiomyopathy ventricular tachyarrhythmia can be a predecessor of progressive heart failure. In one study in patients with ICDs, only 15% of all patients survived 4 years without a cluster of ventricular tachyarrhythmia.[81]

There are two completed prospective studies in patients with nonischemic cardiomyopathy without prior arrhythmias and one in patients with asymptomatic nonsustained ventricular tachycardias. The studies in patients without prior arrhythmias (Cardiomyopathy Trial [CAT][43] and Defibrillators in Nonischemic Cardiomyopathy Treatment Evaluation [DEFINITE])[82] yielded a little conflicting results. CAT was a pilot study in patients with a recently (<9 months) diagnosed nonischemic dilated cardiomyopathy (EF < 30%) that included 102 patients.[43] Patients were randomized to ICD therapy or no antiarrhythmic drug therapy. The primary endpoint of CAT was total mortality after 2 years. In contrast to the investigators' expectations, the total mortality after 2 years was only 8% to 9% in both groups. The study was terminated as more than 1300 patients would have been needed for a significant difference between groups. In the first 2 years after inclusion into the study, there was not a single case of sudden death in the control group. In the ICD group, there were 11 patients with a ventricular tachycardia of more than 200 bpm. All tachycardias were terminated by the implanted devices. Nevertheless, after 5 years only 50% of those patients with appropriate ICD discharges survived in contrast to 85% of the patients without appropriate ICD discharges. This finding is in analogy to the finding of an association between appropriate ICD discharges and death from progressive heart failure.[81]

The findings of the yet unpublished DEFINITE trial are in contrast to the results of the CAT trial. DEFINITE was the first large-scale trial investigating the use of ICDs for the primary prevention of sudden cardiac death (SCD) in patients with nonischemic dilated cardiomyopathy. DEFINITE[83] enrolled a total of 458 patients with nonischemic dilated cardiomyopathy, LV dysfunction (ejection fraction ≤35%), NYHA class I-III heart failure, and spontaneous ventricular arrhythmia (premature ventricular complexes or nonsustained ventricular tachycardia [VT]). Patients with unexplained syncope within

6 months, prior cardiac arrest or VT > 15 beats at a rate ≥ 120 bpm, or those on amiodarone treatment for ventricular arrhythmias were excluded from the study. Patients were randomized to drug therapy with beta-blockers and ACE inhibitors (if tolerated) ($n = 229$) or drug therapy plus an ICD ($n = 229$). All patients in the ICD arm received a single-chamber ICD, which was set at a ventricular fibrillation (VF) detection zone of 180 bpm and was programmed for back-up VVI pacing at 40 bpm. The mean LV ejection fraction was 21% and the mean age was 58.4 years. Mean follow-up was 26 months.

The study's primary endpoint was total mortality; the secondary endpoint was arrhythmic death. In designing the trial, investigators estimated that total 2-year mortality in the control group would be 15% and that use of an ICD would result in a 50% reduction in mortality. The study was designed for termination after the 56th death, which occurred in January 2003.

Of the 56 total deaths, 33 deaths occurred in the drug-only group and 23 deaths occurred in the ICD group. Both total mortality and arrhythmic mortality in the drug-only group were lower than investigators expected, reaching 13.8% and 33%, respectively. *Total mortality* observed in the ICD treatment group was 8.1%, a result that did not reach statistical significance when compared with control ($P = 0.06$), although there was a clear trend toward a benefit. The absolute mortality benefit in the ICD group was 5.7% at 2 years and the relative risk reduction was 34%, which fell considerably short of the trial's goal. ICDs were associated with a significantly lower rate of *arrhythmic death*, the study's secondary endpoint. Of the 56 deaths, 14 were classified as arrhythmic in nature; 11 patients on drug therapy alone died of arrhythmia during the follow-up period, compared with three in the ICD group.

Use of an ICD was associated with a 74% relative reduction in arrhythmic death ($P = 0.01$).

Subgroup analyses uncovered that patients with class III heart failure who received an ICD ($n = 47$) had a 67% relative risk reduction in all-cause mortality compared with those who received drug therapy alone ($n = 49$), and these results were highly significant (13% versus 33%, respectively; $P = 0.009$).

Very recently, first results of the Sudden Cardiac Death in Heart Failure Trial (SCD-HeFT), a 2521-patient study evaluating the use of ICDs and drug therapy (with amiodarone) in patients with class II or III heart failure with an ejection fraction ≤ 0.35 have been presented. Mortality in the placebo arm was 7.2% per year over a 5-year period. There was no difference between patients treated with amiodarone or with placebo. However, prophylactic ICD implantation resulted in a 23% reduction of total mortality without differences between ischemic and nonischemic etiology of the heart failure. SCD-HeFT was the first large scale trial of ICD therapy in a heart failure population and will undubitably have a large impact on further indications for ICD implantation.[78]

Non-sustained ventricular tachycardias are a well-accepted risk factor in patients with coronary artery disease. As mentioned above, ICD therapy has been shown to be beneficial in patients with impaired left ventricular function and nonsustained ventricular tachycardias in the MADIT and the MUSTT trials.[2,47] Accordingly, the hypothesis that ICD therapy would be superior to antiarrhythmic drug therapy also in patients with nonischemic dilated cardiomyopathy and nonsustained ventricular tachycardias was tested in the AMIOVIRT study.[40] In this study, 103 patients with nonischemic dilated cardiomyopathy, left ventricular ejection fraction $\leq 35\%$, and asymptomatic non-sustained VT were randomized to receive either amiodarone or an ICD. The primary end-point was total mortality. The study was stopped because of the unexpectedly low total mortality in both arms. The percentage of patients surviving at one year (90% vs. 96%) and three years (88% versus 87%) in the amiodarone and ICD groups, respectively, were not statistically different ($p = 0.8$). As there was no true placebo group in this study, it cannot be clarified whether non-sustained VT is not useful as a risk predictor in nonischemic dilated cardiomyopathy or whether amiodarone is highly efficient in this patient cohort. The latter had retrospectively been suggested by the CHF-STAT trial where amiodarone proved to be more effective in nonischemic versus ischemic patients.[84] However, in a prospective registry by Grimm et al.[85] including 343 patients with idiopathic dilated cardiomyopathy, only reduced LV ejection fraction and lack of beta-blocker therapy were predictors of an increased arrhythmic risk. Signal-averaged ECG, QTc dispersion, heart rate variability, baroreflex sensitivity, and microvolt TWA did not predict arrhythmia risk and non-sustained ventricular tachycardia on Holter was associated only with a trend toward higher arrhythmia risk. In contrast to these findings, patients with non-sustained VT in the CAT trial had a markedly increased total mortality rate with only 63% surviving after 6 years compared to 77% of the patients without non-sustained VT. However, in CAT, even in this subgroup, there was no benefit from ICD implantation. In patients with nonischemic dilated cardiomyopathy, nonsustained VT seems to be more a marker for increased total mortality than for a high arrhythmic risk.

The findings by Grimm et al.[85] that among others, microvolt TWA did not predict arrhythmia risk is in contrast with the findings of a similar study by Hohnloser et al.[86] in 137 patients with idiopathic dilated cardiomyopathy who found that microvolt-level TWA is a powerful independent predictor of ventricular tachyarrhythmic events.

In the yet unpublished COMPANION trial, a total of 1634 NYHA class III/IV heart failure patients with a QRS interval of >120 ms, PR interval >150 ms, and a left ventricular ejection fraction ≤35% were enrolled. They were treated with optimal pharmacologic therapy, a regimen that consisted of beta-blockers, diuretics as needed, angiotensin-converting enzyme inhibitors or angiotensin receptor blockers, spironolactone, and/or digoxin. Patients were then randomized in a 1:2:2 ratio to receive either optimal pharmacologic therapy alone (OPT) or in combination with resynchronization therapy (CRT), or in combination with resynchronization therapy and a defibrillator (CRT-D). They were followed for a period of 12 months. The study's primary endpoint was a composite of all-cause mortality and hospitalization. Secondary endpoints included separate analyses of all-cause mortality, cardiac morbidity, and exercise performance.

Both the CRT and CRT-D groups had statistically significant (19%) reductions in the primary endpoint of combined all-cause hospitalization and all-cause mortality when compared with OPT. The similarity between the two device arms suggests that the treatment effect related to this endpoint was due to the impact of CRT and was not heavily influenced by the addition of the implantable defibrillator. CRT-D had a much greater effect on the secondary endpoint of all-cause mortality than CRT alone, demonstrating a highly significant, 43.4% reduction in all-cause mortality, and this effect was observable early on in the follow-up period. By comparison, the CRT group achieved a 23.9% reduction (nonsignificant) in all-cause mortality, which was not observable until late in the follow-up period. Additionally, investigators reported that CRT and CRT-D were each associated with a decrease in combined all-cause mortality and heart failure hospitalization. Subgroup analysis revealed a uniform mortality treatment effect for all patient subgroups and no obvious difference in mortality between patients with ischemic and nonischemic cardiomyopathy.

Thus, prophylactic ICD implantation might be indicated especially in those patients with nonischemic dilated cardiomyopathy, who also receive an optimal treatment for heart failure, which might be able to decouple myocardial function and arrhythmic risk.

Brugada Syndrome

Brugada syndrome was first described as a new clinical entity in 1992.[87] The electrocardiographic features of the syndrome include: (1) an accentuated J wave appearing in the right precordial leads (V1-V3) and taking the form of an ST segment elevation, often followed by a negative T-wave; (2) very closely coupled ventricular extrasystoles; and (3) rapid polymorphic ventricular tachycardia, which at times may be indistinguishable from ventricular fibrillation. Three types of repolarization patterns are recognized.[88] The ECG sign of Brugada syndrome is dynamic and often concealed, but can be unmasked by potent sodium channel blockers such as flecainide (2 mg/kg body weight; max 150 mg; in 10 min), ajmalin (1 mg/kg body weight; 10 mg/min), or procainamide (10 mg/kg body weight; 100 mg/min).[88–90] The typical ECG changes can also be unmasked by vagotonic agents, beta-blockers, alcohol intoxication, fever, and a variety of other drugs (Figures 5 and 6).[91–93]

	Type 1	Type 2	Type 3
J-wave amplitude	≥ 2 mm	≥ 2 mm	≥ 2 mm
T-wave	Negative	Positive or biphasic	Positive
ST-T configuration	Coved type	Saddle back	Saddle back
ST segment (terminal portion)	Gradually descending	Elevated ≥ 1 mm	Elevated < 1 mm

1 mm= 0.1 mV ;

the terminal portion of the ST-segment refers to the latter half of the ST-segment

Figure 5. ST segment abnormalities in leads V1-V3.[88])

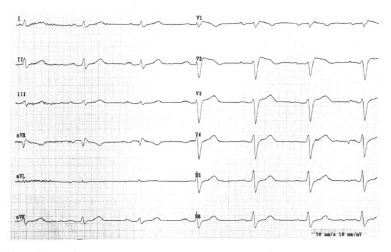

Figure 6. Typical ECG changes of Brugada syndrome (Type 1).

Secondary prevention of cardiac arrest in patients with
Brugada syndrome
It is well accepted that patients with Brugada syndrome
once they have survived an episode of ventricular fibrillation should be treated with an ICD. Therefore, it is very
unlikely that in North America or Western Europe a trial
comparing ICD therapy to any other therapy will be con-
ducted in the foreseeable future.

Brugada syndrome seems to be identical to the Sudden Unexplained Death Syndrome (SUDS) in young,
healthy, Southeast Asian men.[94] In the latter entity, defibrillator implantation was compared to beta-blocker
therapy in a small randomized trial of 86 patients.[44] There
were seven deaths (18%) in the beta-blocker group and
no deaths in the ICD group, but there were a total of
12 ICD patients receiving ICD discharges due to recurrent VF. Thus, this prospective randomized trial provides
strong arguments for ICD implantation in these patients.
It should be noted that the use of beta-blockers in the control group might possibly have increased the rate of VF recurrences as beta-blockers are among the drugs that can
unmask the typical ECG changes observed in Brugada
syndrome.

From experiments in perfused wedges of canine
right ventricle there is evidence that quinidine might
be an effective pharmacological treatment for Brugada
syndrome.[95] Quinidine has also been suggested as an effective therapy for Brugada syndrome by Belhassen.[30] As
no data from randomized trials of ICD versus quinidine
are available, ICD therapy, which is very effective in the
prevention of a catastrophic outcome of a tachyarrhythmic episode, has to be considered as therapy of first choice.
Risk stratifiers, such as inducibility at programmed ventricular stimulation, do not play a role in patients with
aborted sudden death.

Primary prevention of sudden death in patients with the Brugada ECG pattern
The prognosis and approach in patients with an ECG diagnostic of Brugada syndrome but without a previous history of sudden cardiac death are controversial. The largest series so far has been published by Brugada et al.[96] They studied a total of 547 patients with an ECG diagnostic of Brugada syndrome and no previous cardiac arrest. The diagnostic ECG was spontaneously present in 391 patients. In the remaining 156 individuals, the abnormal ECG was noted only after the administration of an antiarrhythmic drug. One hundred twenty-four patients had suffered from at least one episode of syncope. During programmed ventricular stimulation, a sustained ventricular arrhythmia was induced in 163 of 408 patients. During a mean follow-up of 24 ± 32 months, 45 patients (8%) suffered sudden death or documented ventricular fibrillation. Multivariate analysis identified the inducibility of a sustained ventricular arrhythmia ($P < 0.0001$) and a history of syncope ($P < 0.01$) as predictors of events. Logistic regression analysis showed that a patient with a spontaneously abnormal ECG, a previous history of syncope, and inducible sustained ventricular arrhythmias had a probability of 27.2% of suffering an event during follow up.

In contrast to these findings, Gasparini et al.[97] found the reproducibility of electrophysiological studies in Brugada syndrome low, and Eckardt et al. found that the extent of inducibility was dependent on the stimulation protocol used.[98] Priori et al.[99] analyzed 200 patients (152 men, 48 women) and failed to demonstrate an association between inducibility at programmed electrical stimulation and spontaneous occurrence of ventricular fibrillation. In their analysis, after adjusting for sex, family history of sudden death, and SCN5A mutations, the combined presence of a spontaneous ST-segment elevation in

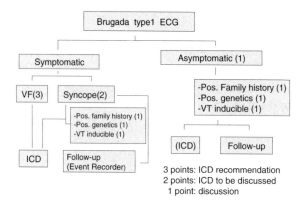

Figure 7. Approach to patients with Brugada syndrome.

leads V1 through V3 and the history of syncope identified subjects at risk of cardiac arrest (hazard ratio, 6.4; 95% CI, 1.9 to 21; $P < 0.002$). Both groups state that an extended follow-up is needed before firm conclusions about natural history, risk of sudden death, and response to therapy in patients with Brugada syndrome can be drawn. Until then, an individualized approach to each patient is necessary. The current approach at our institution is depicted in the accompanying figure (see Figure 7).

Hypertrophic Cardiomyopathy

Hypertrophic cardiomyopathy is an inherited cardiac disease with a heterogeneous presentation and a diverse natural history. The disease is often familial, with autosomal-dominant transmission. More than 150 different mutations in 11 genes that encode sarcomeric or other muscular proteins have been described.[100–103] The disease affects sarcomeric proteins, resulting in small vessel disease, myocyte and myofibrillar disorganization, and fibrosis with or without myocardial hypertrophy. The classical pattern of asymmetric septal hypertrophy may be accompanied by systolic anterior movement of the mitral valve (SAM) and dynamic left ventricular outflow tract obstruction that can cause exertional symptoms. The disease is usually benign in its clinical course, but <5% of the patients exhibit progressive deterioration in left ventricular function and dilatation.[104]

Sudden death resulting from ventricular fibrillation has been recognized as a prominent cause of death in patients with hypertrophic cardiomyopathy that occurs not uncommonly in asymptomatic patients. SCD is most frequent in adolescents and young adults but can also occur during midlife or beyond. It occurs most often during mild exertion, sedentary activities or sleep; vigorous exertion is a well-known trigger.

Various treatment modalities including beta-blockers, calcium channel antagonists, disopyramide, myectomy, alcohol septal ablation, and dual chamber pacing have been proposed for treatment of obstruction.[105] All patients with hypertrophic cardiomyopathy should also undergo risk stratification for sudden cardiac death.

Secondary prevention of cardiac arrest or sustained ventricular tachycardias in hypertrophic cardiomyopathy
Historically, the prophylactic management was limited to pharmacologic treatment with beta-blockers and antiarrhythmic drugs, most recently predominantly with amiodarone.[106] However, prospective data to support this recommendation have never been obtained. The efficacy of implantable defibrillators for terminating life-threatening ventricular tachyarrhythmia has been widely accepted. However, despite the widespread use of ICDs in

patients with coronary artery disease, there has been little application of devices to patients with hypertrophic cardiomyopathy. In a small series of patients with HCM and resuscitated VF, Elliott et al. found a high recurrence rate both, in patients treated with amiodarone or with a defibrillator.[107] The largest series so far has been published by Maron and coworkers. In a retrospective registry including 43 patients who were treated with an ICD for secondary prevention of sudden cardiac arrest or sustained ventricular tachycardia, they found recurrences in 11% per year.[108] Sixty percent of those who experienced appropriate ICD interventions had multiple episodes. This rate was about twice as high as in 85 patients treated prophylactically (i.e., for primary prevention) with an ICD. Not surprisingly, ICDs were extremely effective in terminating such tachyarrhythmias.

Primary prevention of sudden death in hypertrophic cardiomyopathy

Risk stratification. The registry data presented by Maron et al.,[108] although retrospective, are the first in a large group of HCM patients. The 85 patients receiving ICDs solely for primary prevention showed an appropriate intervention rate of 5% per year. High risk leading to the implantation of the devices was based on the identification of one or more risk factors: family history of hypertrophic cardiomyopathy-related sudden death, exertional syncope, multiple repetitive or prolonged nonsustained ventricular tachycardia on ambulatory ECG, or extreme left ventricular hypertrophy (≥30 mm). The presence or absence of LV outflow tract obstruction was not a risk factor for sudden death. It should be noted that the complication rate for ICD therapy was substantial in this population (25%). In a study by Montserrat et al., a correlation between nonsustained ventricular tachycardia and risk of sudden death was found in young patients, not so much in older patients.[109] The relation between the frequency, duration, and rate of nonsustained VT episodes could not be demonstrated. The implication of that retrospective study in 531 patients was that prophylactic ICD implantation is justified when nonsustained VTs occur in young patients. In contrast, nonsustained VT in older patients does not justify ICD therapy when it occurs without other risk factors, such as severe LV hypertrophy, history of presyncope or syncope, or abnormal blood pressure response to exercise.[110]

The risk markers recognized in the multicenter ICD registry[108] have been included in a consensus document by an ACC/ESC expert group (see Table 2).[105]

Most of the clinical markers of sudden cardiac death risk are limited by a relatively low positive predictive value. However, absence of risk factors identifies a large proportion of patients who can be reassured of having a low risk of sudden death. On the other side, it seems

Table 2. *Risk factors for sudden cardiac death in HOCM*[105]

Major
- Cardiac arrest (ventricular fibrillation)
- Spontaneous sustained ventricular fibrillation
- Family history of premature sudden death
- Unexplained syncope
- LV thickness greater than or equal to 30 mm
- Abnormal exercise blood pressure
- Nonsustained ventricular tachycardia (Holter)

Possible in individual patients
- Atrial fibrillation
- Myocardial ischemia
- Left ventricular outflow obstruction
- High-risk mutation
- Intense (competitive) physical exertion

possible to identify most high-risk patients by noninvasive clinical markers and only a small minority of those patients who die suddenly are without any of the currently acknowledged risk markers.[111]

The highest risk has been associated with the following: (1) prior cardiac arrest or spontaneously occurring and sustained VT, (2) family history of a premature HCM-related sudden cardiac death in a close relative or in multiple relatives, (3) identification of a high-risk mutant gene, (4) unexplained syncope, particularly in young patients or when exertional or recurrent, (5) nonsustained VT (≥ 3 beats of at least 120 bpm), (6) abnormal blood pressure response during upright exercise, which is attenuated or hypotensive, indicative of hemodynamic instability, and of greater predictive value in patients <50 years old or if hypotensive, (7) extreme left ventricular hypertrophy with a maximum wall thickness of ≥ 30 mm, particularly in adolescents and young adults.[105] Although the concept of extreme hypertrophy as a sole risk factor is not unequivocally resolved, it is currently considered sufficient to justify a recommendation for a prophylactic ICD implantation, especially in younger patients.[105,111–113]

It has been proposed that some genetic defects are associated with a higher incidence of premature death whereas other mutations convey a more favorable prognosis. This finding formed the basis for the aspiration of formulating a genotype risk stratification strategy. However, by analyzing a large consecutively accessed cohort of unrelated individuals, it has been shown that mutations previously described as "benign" or "malignant" are particularly uncommon in the HCM population and are also of uncertain prognostic significance.[114,115]

Currently, it is unknown whether the grouping of mutations by functional domain may improve gene-based

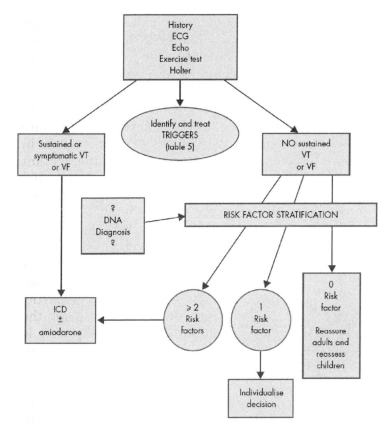

Figure 8. Algorithm for risk stratification and prevention of sudden death.[104]

risk stratification.[116,117] In clinical practice, the search for mutations to improve risk stratification has no role (see Figure 8).

Treatment. There is no evidence that medical treatment strategies using drugs such as beta-blockers, verapamil, or class I antiarrhythmics reduce the risk of sudden cardiac death. Amiodarone has been suggested to re-duce sudden death rate[106,118] although this assumption is based only on retrospective data. In addition, amiodarone may not be tolerated due to its potential toxicity over long periods incurred by young patients. When the risk level for sudden cardiac death is judged by contemporary criteria to be unacceptably high and deserving of intervention, the ICD is the most effective and reliable treatment option available.

In the registry data presented by Maron et al.,[108] the 85 patients receiving ICDs solely for primary prevention showed an appropriate intervention rate of 5% per year. It is of interest that ICD often remained dormant for prolonged periods before discharging (up to 9 years), emphasizing the unpredictable timing of sudden cardiac death events in this disease, the potentially long risk period, and the requirement for extended follow-up periods in HCM studies.

The ACC/AHA 2002 guidelines have designated the ICD for primary prevention of sudden cardiac death as a class IIb indication.

Long QT Syndrome

The long QT syndrome (LQTS) is characterized by the appearance of long QT intervals in the ECG, an atypical ventricular tachycardia known as torsade de pointes (TdP), and a high risk for sudden cardiac death.[119–122] The congenital long QT syndrome is the best known primary electrical disorder of the heart. Meanwhile, more than 250 mutations in seven genes (LQTS 1-7) have been described. The identification of LQTS genes has provided tremendous new insights into our understanding of normal cardiac electrophysiology and its perturbation in a

Table 3. *Relation between genotype and phenotype in LQTS*

	LQT1	LQT2	LQT3
Prevalence	42	45	8
Trigger	Exercise	Sudden noise	Rest/sleep
Age at 1st event	9	12	16
Mortality/event (%)	4	4	20
β-Blocker	+++	++	+

wide range of conditions associated with sudden death (see Table 3). In 30% to 40% of all patients with LQTS, no gene defect can be found pointing toward a large heterogeneity of gene loci. Associations between genotype and phenotype have been investigated based on the international LQTS registry, which was started already in 1979. In a recent study,[123] data from 533 genotyped index patients (243 LQT1, 209 LQT2, 81 LQT3) and 1842 family members were analyzed. Mortality was highest in patients with LQT3 followed by male patients with LQT1 and LQT2 and female patients with LQT1 and LQT2. However, arrhythmic events occurred more frequently in LQT1 and LQT2. Priori et al.[124] presented a scheme for risk stratification based on an analysis of 647 patients. High risk was considered in patients with LQT1 and QTc > 500 ms$^{1/2}$ and in male patients with LQT2 or LQT3 and QTC > 500 ms$^{1/2}$. High-risk patients should be treated prophylactically using beta-blockers[125] although the effect is less beneficial in patients with LQT1 (Figure 9).[126]

The term "acquired LQTS" is reserved for a syndrome similar to the congenital form but caused by exposure to drugs that prolong the duration of the ventricular action potential or to QT prolongation secondary to bradycardia or an electrolyte imbalance. Prophylactic

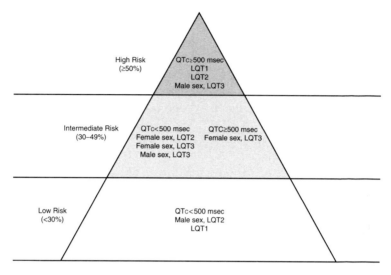

Figure 9. Risk stratification in patients with long QT syndrome.[124]

ICD implantation is not necessary for patients with an acquired LQTS. It should be noted that other disease states such as hypertrophic or dilated cardiomyopathy go along with a reduced repolarization reserve as well.

Results of ICD therapy in patients with the long QT syndrome
There is only limited information available on the impact of ICD therapy in patients with congenital long QT syndrome. In clinical practice, the decision for prophylactic ICD implantation is not based on gene analysis. Usually, prophylactic ICD implantation is considered indicated in patients experiencing syncopes despite betablocker therapy or in patients with syncope and with a family history of sudden death. For these patient cohorts, a benefit from ICD implantation has been suggested by retrospective analyses. Zareba et al.[127] described a

comparison between 73 LQTS patients treated with ICDs because of cardiac arrest ($n = 54$) or recurrent syncope despite beta-blocker therapy ($n = 19$) to 161 LQTS patients who had similar indications (89 indications of cardiac arrest and 72 indications of recurrent syncope despite beta-blocker therapy) but did not receive ICDs. There was 1 (1.3%) death in 73 ICD patients followed for an average of 3 years, whereas there were 26 deaths (16%) in non-ICD patients during mean 8-year follow-up ($P = 0.07$ from log rank test from Kaplan-Meier curves). However, this analysis was questioned by Viskin[128] who pointed out that after exclusion of the patients who died within 1 month after inclusion and therefore likely from residuals of their first aborted sudden death, the difference between both groups were only marginal. Both agreed that a long-term prospective study is needed to determine the benefit of ICD therapy in LQTS patients.

The ACC/AHA 2002 guidelines have designated the ICD for primary prevention of SCD as a class IIb indication (Figure 10).

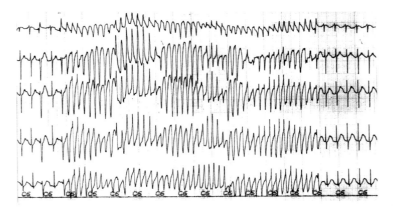

Figure 10. Torsade de pointes.

Short QT Syndrome

Very recently, a new syndrome associated with sudden cardiac death in otherwise healthy patients with structurally normal hearts has been described, the short QT syndrome.[129–130] Six patients from two European families were extensively tested by noninvasive and invasive methods. Mean QT intervals were 252 ± 13 ms (QTc 287 ± 13 ms). In four patients, electrophysiological studies were performed revealing short atrial and ventricular refractory periods in all and increased ventricular vulnerability to fibrillation in three of four patients.[129,130] In two of the affected families, two different missense mutations were described resulting in the same amino acid change of the cardiac IKr channel HERG (KCNH2). The mutations dramatically increase IKr, leading to a heterogeneous abbreviation of action potential duration and refractoriness, and reducing the affinity of the channels to IKr blockers.[131] In five patients, defibrillators were implanted as the physicians thought that ICD treatment was the only therapeutic option.[132] Despite normal sensing behavior during intraoperative and postoperative device testing, three of five patients experienced inappropriate shock therapies for T wave oversensing 30 ± 26 days after implantation. Nothing is known about the frequency of appropriate shocks. However, given a family history of sudden cardiac death, in patients with the short QT syndrome prophylactic ICD implantation might be considered appropriate. In the current guidelines, the short QT syndrome is not mentioned, but as a familial or inherited condition with a high risk of SCD, it is a class IIb indication for ICD implantation.

Arrhythmogenic Right Ventricular Cardiomyopathy

Arrhythmogenic right ventricular dysplasia/cardio-myopathy (ARVD/C) was first described in 1982[133] and since then has been diagnosed with increased frequency. It has been reported to account for 3% to 10% of unexplained sudden cardiac death under the age of 65 years.[134] Mutations in eight genetic loci have been associated with the disease,[100] and three different genes have been identified, coding for ryanodine receptor (RyR2),[135] plakoglobin (JUP),[136] and desmoplakin.[137] There are large variations in the clinical presentation of patients with ARVD/C ranging from asymptomatic ventricular ectopy usually of left bundle branch block morphology to aborted sudden death. Structural changes might be minimal and therefore difficult to identify. Usually, a whole series of diagnostic tests has to be used for the diagnosis of ARVD/C or its exclusion (Table 4).[138]

At present, information is limited regarding the clinical course of ARVD/C even in patients with overt disease and significant ventricular arrhythmias, and even less is known about asymptomatic, affected family members. There is also incomplete knowledge of factors that might permit accurate risk stratification. Therefore, treatment for patients diagnosed with ARVD/C is empirical, and the decision which patient should be treated with a defibrillator must be individualized as no precise guidelines exist to select patients who should be treated with beta-blockers, antiarrhythmic drugs, or an ICD. Patients with well-tolerated and non-life-threatening ventricular arrhythmias are usually treated empirically with antiarrhythmic drugs, including amiodarone, sotalol, beta-blockers, flecainide, and propafenone, alone or in

Table 4. *Task force criteria for diagnosis of right ventricular dysplasia/cardiomyopathy*

---

1. Global and/or regional dysfunction and structural alterations
   Major
   • Severe dilatation and reduction of right ventricular ejection fraction with no (or only mild) LV involvement
   • Localized right ventricular aneurysms (akinetic or dyskinetic areas with diastolic bulging)
   • Severe segmental dilatation of the right ventricle
   Minor
   • Mild global right ventricular dilatation and/or ejection fraction reduction with normal left ventricle
   • Mild segmental dilatation of the right ventricle
   • Regional right ventricular hypokinesia
2. Tissue characterization of wall
   Major
   • Fibrofatty replacement of myocardium on endomyocardial biopsy
3. Repolarization abnormalities
   Minor
   • Inverted T waves in right precordial leads (V2 and V3) in people aged >12 years, in the absence of right bundle branch block
4. Depolarization/conduction abnormalities
   Major
   • Epsilon waves or localized prolongation (>110 ms) of the QRS complex in right precordial leads (V1-V3)
   Minor
   • Late potentials (signal-averaged ECG)
5. Arrhythmias
   Minor
   • Left bundle branch block type ventricular tachycardia (sustained and nonsustained) by ECG, Holter, or exercise testing
   • Frequent ventricular extrasystoles (>1000/24 hours) (Holter)
6. Family history
   Major
   • Familial disease confirmed at necropsy or surgery
   Minor
   • Family history of premature sudden death (<35 years) due to suspected right ventricular dysplasia
   • Familial history (clinical diagnosis based on present criteria

---

The diagnosis of ARVD/C would be fulfilled by the presence of 2 major, 1 major plus 2 minor, or 4 minor criteria from different groups.[138,139]

combination.[140,141] Implantable defibrillators are usually reserved for patients with life-threatening ventricular arrhythmias in whom drug therapy is either ineffective or undesirable.[142-144] Recently, a series of 132 patients from 23 hospitals in Northern Italy and the United States was published, which was by far the largest published series so far.[145] Implant indications were a history of cardiac arrest in 13 patients (10%), sustained ventricular tachycardia in 82 (62%), syncope in 21 (16%), nonsustained ventricular tachycardia in 12 (9%), and a family history of sudden death in 4 patients (3%). During a mean follow-up of 39 $\pm$ 25 months, 64 patients (48%) had appropriate ICD interventions, 21 (16%) had inappropriate interventions, and 19 (14%) had ICD-related complications. Four patients (3%) died, and 32 (24%) experienced ventricular fibrillation/flutter that in all likelihood would have been fatal in the absence of the device. At 36 months, the actual patient survival rate was 96% compared with the ventricular fibrillation/flutter-free survival rate of 72% ($P < 0.001$).

Programmed ventricular stimulation was of limited value in identifying patients at risk of tachyarrhythmias during the follow-up (positive predictive value 49%, negative predictive value 54%). Patients who received implants because of ventricular tachycardia without hemodynamic compromise had a significantly lower incidence of ventricular fibrillation/flutter (log rank = 0.01). History of cardiac arrest or ventricular tachycardia with hemodynamic compromise, younger age, and left ventricular involvement were independent predictors of ventricular fibrillation/flutter. Wichter et al.[146] found in a series of 60 patients in a single center, which during a mean follow-up of 80 $\pm$ 43 months, had an event-free rate after 5 years and was only 26% for ventricular tachycardias and 59% for potentially fatal ventricular tachycardias with a rate

>240 bpm. Extensive right ventricular dysfunction was identified as a predictor for appropriate ICD discharges. Prospective and controlled studies assessing clinical markers are needed to get a clearer picture of factors that might predict the occurrence of life-threatening ventricular arrhythmias.

Catecholamine- or Exercise-Induced Polymorphic Ventricular Tachycardia

Catecholaminergic polymorphic ventricular tachycardia (CPVT) is a clinically and genetically heterogeneous disease manifesting with a spectrum of polymorphic arrhythmias. It is characterized by episodes of syncope, seizures, or sudden death in response to physiological or emotional stress. This disease with autosomal dominant inheritance was first described as manifesting in a Bedouin tribe from Israel[147] but was also found in other populations.[148–150] Around 40% to 60% of the patients with catecholaminergic polymorphic ventricular tachycardia (CPVT) carry mutations in the cardiac ryanodine receptor gene (RyR2)[151] or in the calsequestrin 2 gene (CASQ2).[152] Documented arrhythmias included bidirectional ventricular tachycardia, polymorphic ventricular tachycardia, and in rare patients catecholaminergic idiopathic ventricular fibrillation. The majority of patients responds favorably to treatment with beta-blockers,[147,151] but in 30% of patients an implantable defibrillator may be required (Figure 11).[151]

Other Patients Believed at High Risk

Defibrillators as a bridge to heart transplantation
About 20% of the patients requiring heart transplantation die awaiting a donor organ. The incidence of sudden

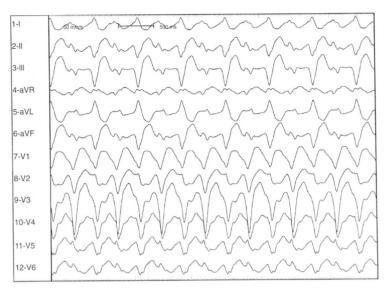

Figure 11. Bidirectional tachycardia in a patient with a history of cardiac arrest and exercise-related polymorphic VT.

death in this patient cohort is substantial. ICDs have been associated with a lower risk of sudden death in these patients,[153,154] but the effect on total mortality is diluted by the competing risk of dying from progressive heart failure. In a study by Sweeney et al.[154] in 291 patients referred for evaluation of heart transplantation, ICD therapy reduced the rate of sudden death compared to the group without antiarrhythmic treatment from 16% to 9%, but total mortality did not differ. In a similar study of 228 consecutive heart transplant candidates on the waiting list published by Grimm et al.,[153] the absence of an implantable cardioverter defibrillator was only a marginally significant predictor of mortality ($P = 0.079$). However, the absence of an implantable cardioverter defibrillator was a powerful predictor of mortality for a subgroup of

134 patients with high-grade ventricular arrhythmias on Holter electrocardiography and for a subgroup of 58 survivors of sudden cardiac death.

Of the 60 selected heart transplant candidates with a history of successful resuscitation by external electric defibrillation for spontaneous, syncopal ventricular tachyarrhythmia, 30 received an ICD, whereas 30 patients lacked ICD therapy for various non-medical reasons. Survival on the waiting list was significantly improved by ICD therapy; only 1 surviving of the 30 ICD patients but 7 of the 30 non-ICD patients died on the waiting list. Prospective randomized trials in this patient cohort have not yet been published. Currently, being a candidate for heart transplantation alone does not qualify for prophylactic ICD implantation. However, a significant proportion of the patients on the waiting list for heart transplantation would also fulfill the criteria for entry into the MADIT II trial, thus having a class IIa indication according to current guidelines.

Cardiac Resynchronization Therapy (CRT)

Biventricular pacing has emerged as a new therapy for patients, with class III or IV heart failure despite optimized drug therapy, who are in sinus rhythm and have a prolonged QRS duration. Early studies using a crossover design proved the concept that biventricular pacing with the LV electrode at the free lateral wall could improve symptoms of heart failure and increase exercise tolerance.[155,156]

More recently, a larger study was done, the Miracle trial, which included 453 patients with class III or IV heart failure associated with an ejection fraction $\leq 35\%$

and a QRS interval of ≥130 ms. Patients assigned to CRT experienced a significant improvement in the distance walked in 6 minutes (+39 versus +10 m), functional class (P < 0.001), quality of life (−18.0 versus −9.0 points), which were the primary endpoints. In addition, ejection fraction increased by +4.6% versus −0.2%, and fewer CRT patients required hospitalization (8% versus 15%) for the treatment of heart failure. However, device implantation was associated with significant morbidity and mortality: It was unsuccessful in 8% of patients and was complicated by refractory hypotension, bradycardia, or asystole in four patients (two of whom died) and by perforation of the coronary sinus requiring pericardiocentesis in two others.[157]

Early on, the question has been posed whether biventricular pacing has proarrhythmic or antiarrhythmic effects. There are only very few reports of proarrhythmia in the literature.[158] A small cross-over study showed a reduction of appropriate ICD interventions during biventricular pacing compared to right-ventricular pacing[159] and in another very small study, biventricular pacing reduced the number of ventricular ectopic beats and runs of non-sustained ventricular tachycardia.[160] In a meta-analysis of four published trials on resynchronization therapy including 1634 patients, cardiac resynchronization had no clear impact on ventricular tachycardia or ventricular fibrillation (odds ratio, 0.92).[161]

Very recently, results of the COMPANION trial (Comparison of Medical Therapy, Pacing, and Defibrillation in Chronic Heart Failure) have been presented but not yet been published. COMPANION enrolled a total of 1634 NYHA class III/IV heart failure patients with a QRS interval of >120 ms, a PR interval >150 ms, and a left ventricular ejection fraction ≤35% who were treated with optimal pharmacologic therapy, a regimen that consisted of beta-blockers, diuretics as needed, angiotensin-converting enzyme inhibitors or angiotensin receptor blockers, spironolactone, and/or digoxin. Patients were randomized in a 1:2:2 ratio to receive either optimal medical therapy alone or in combination with biventricular pacing or in combination with biventricular pacing plus defibrillation backup. Patients were followed for a period of 12 months. The study's primary endpoint was a composite of all-cause mortality and hospitalization. Secondary endpoints included separate analyses of all-cause mortality, cardiac morbidity, and exercise performance. The study showed that patients who received a combination of biventricular pacing and defibrillation backup had a higher benefit and a lower mortality rate compared to patients who were treated with biventricular pacing alone. And the latter patient group had a better outcome than those patients who were treated only with optimized drug therapy. Preliminary analysis failed to show a differential benefit for patients with coronary artery disease versus patients with idiopathic dilated cardiomyopathy. It is very likely that the inclusion criteria tested in COMPANION will become a class IIa indication for the implantation of a defibrillator/biventricular pacemaker in the next rounds of guidelines for ICD implantation.

A point to note is that whereas this new therapy is now called cardiac resynchronization therapy, a proof of desynchronization of both ventricles or of septum and lateral wall of the left ventricle was not required to enter the study. QRS width was used as a surrogate for desynchronization. While it is very likely that the vast majority of patients with a QRS > 150 ms (this was required to be included into the older studies of biventricular pacing)

Table 5. *Indications for ICD therapy related to clinical presentation.*

	ACC/AHA 2002[7]	ESC 2001[9]	Comment	References
Cardiac arrest				
• Documented VF or VT not due to a transient or reversible cause	I/A	I/A		1,15–18,23,24,39, 41,65,166–173
• VF or VT resulting from arrhythmias amenable to surgical or catheter ablation; for example, atrial arrhythmias associated with the Wolff-Parkinson-White syndrome, right ventricular outflow tract VT, idiopathic left ventricular tachycardia, or fascicular VT.	III/C	III/C		37,174–177
• Cardiac arrest presumed to be due to VF when electrophysiological testing is precluded by other medical conditions	IIb/C	IIb/C		40,171,178,179
• Ventricular tachyarrhythmias due to a transient or reversible disorder (e.g., AMI, electrolyte imbalance, drugs, or trauma) when correction of the disorder is considered feasible and likely to substantially reduce the risk of recurrent arrhythmia.	III/B			180,181,71

(continued p. 56)

Table 5. *Continued*

	ACC/AHA 2002[7]	ESC 2001[9]	Comment	References
Electrocardiographically documented ventricular tachycardia without cardiac arrest				
• Spontaneous sustained VT in association with structural heart disease	I/B	I/A	In the ESC guidelines, only sustained VT with severe hemodynamic compromise is considered a class I indication Sustained VT without hemodynamic compromise is classified as II/C if LVEF ≤ 40% and III/C if LVEF > 40%	1,15–18,39, 65,166–173
• Spontaneous sustained VT in patients who do not have structural heart disease that is not amenable to other treatments	I/C		This is not mentioned in the ESC guidelines	
• Incessant VT or VF	III/C	III/C		

Non-sustained VT

• Non-sustained VT with coronary disease, prior MI, LV dysfunction, and inducible VF or sustained VT at electrophysiological study that is not suppressible by a class I antiarrhythmic drug.	I/A	I/B	The strict MADIT criteria including demonstration that inducibility cannot be suppressed by class I drugs are not required for ICD implantation according to ESC guidelines.	2,47
• Non-sustained VT with coronary artery disease, prior MI, and LV dysfunction, and inducible sustained VT or VF at electrophysiological study.	IIb/B			
• Severe symptoms (e.g., syncope) attributable to ventricular tachyarrhythmias while awaiting cardiac transplantation.	IIb/C	II/C		153,154

Syncope without documented ventricular tachyarrhythmia

• Syncope of undetermined origin with clinically relevant, hemodynamically significant sustained VT or VF induced at the electrophysiological stage, when drug therapy is ineffective, not tolerated, or not preferred	I/B	I/B or II/C	According to ESC guidelines this is a class I/B indication only if LVEF ≤ 40%, otherwise a class II/C indication	24,65,182

(continued p. 58)

Table 5. *Continued*

	ACC/AHA 2002[7]	ESC 2001[9]	Comment	References
• Syncope of unexplained etiology in association with typical or atypical right bundle-branch block and ST-segment elevations (Brugada syndrome)	IIb/C	II/C		99,183
• Syncope in patients with advanced structural heart disease in which thorough invasive and noninvasive investigation has failed to define a cause	IIb/C	II/C		
• Syncope of undetermined cause in a patient without inducible ventricular tachyarrhythmia and without structural heart disease	III/C	III/C		
Prophylactic indication				
• Patients with LV ejection fraction of less than or equal to 30%, at least one month post myocardial infarction and three months past coronary artery revascularization surgery.	IIa/B	IIa/B	This is stated in the ESC guidelines on prevention of sudden death	42
• Familial or inherited conditions with a high risk for life-threatening ventricular tachyarrhythmias such as long QT syndrome or hypertrophic cardiomyopathy	IIb/B	II/C		

• Family history of unexplained sudden cardiac death in association with typical or atypical right bundle-branch block and ST-segment elevations (Brugada syndrome)	IIb/C	II/C	99,183
• Patients with coronary artery disease with LV dysfunction and prolonged QRS duration in the absence of spontaneous or inducible sustained or non-sustained VT who are undergoing coronary bypass surgery	III/B	III/B	46
General contraindications			
• Significant psychiatric illnesses that may preclude systematic follow-up	III/C	III/C	184,185
• Terminal illnesses with projected life expectancy less than six months	III/C	III/C	
• NYHA class IV drug-refractory congestive heart failure in patients who are not candidates for cardiac transplantation	III/C	III/C	
• Patients who have severe neurological sequelae following cardiac arrest	III/C	III/C	This is not mentioned as a contraindication to ICD therapy in the ACG/AHA guidelines

have some desynchronization, this remains unclear in the patients with a QRS between 120 and 150 ms. Also, the demonstration that the goal of resynchronization was achieved was not done in these studies. More and more evidence emerges that desynchronization can also occur in patients with a narrow QRS complex,[162] although it is still unclear whether the extent of the benefit of resynchronization therapy is the same in this patient cohort.[163] Whether these patients also derive more benefit when resynchronization therapy is combined with defibrillation backup is still unclear. It is noteworthy, however, that those patients who receive resynchronization therapy because of ischemic cardiomyopathy already have a class IIa indication for ICD therapy according to the MADIT II study. It has been shown that the benefit of ICD therapy was greatest in patients with a wide QRS complex, thus underlining the necessity of defibrillation therapy in this part of the patient population that is treated with resynchronization therapy.

Legal Implications of Defibrillator Guidelines

Many respected national or international colleges of physicians, associations, and societies that convene general or specialty groups are developing and publishing guidelines written by recognized experts. These guidelines are developed to aid the practitioner in pursuing the most appropriate health care response for the clinical circumstances of a specific patient. The guidelines from an international society such as the European Society of Cardiology or the World Heart Federation, have no legal territory and have no legal enforcing character.[164] It seems straightforward that the closer the issuing organ is to the recipients, the greater is the chance that the guidelines will be accepted. Guidelines from international organizations may, however, serve as a framework for the issuing of guidelines at a national level, thereby possibly becoming enforceable by the health authorities of that particular country. It is worth noting that guidelines issued by professional medical and/or scientific organizations have no specific legal authority and are in no way legally binding. They may, however, gain an indirect legal character if the courts determine that they represent standard of care for medical practice.

Guidelines cannot be appropriate for all clinical situations. The decision to follow or not to follow a recommendation from a guideline must be made by the physician on an individual basis, taking into account the specific conditions of the patient. Guidelines may be considered as a corridor that helps physicians to separate necessary from unnecessary items. Deviations from guidelines should not be understood as restrictions of therapeutic freedom. Ideally, they should be considered as a chance for orientation in a healthcare system characterized by rationing and rationalization.

This is also accepted in the recent American guidelines for pacemaker and defibrillator implantation.[7] Despite the fact that ICD implantation is considered as indicated (class IIa) in chronic post-myocardial infarction patients with poor left ventricular function, the therapeutic freedom of treating physicians is emphasized. "Although such patients merit consideration of ICD therapy, this approach requires consideration of the patient's overall health and life expectancy. Additional risk stratification studies are needed to better define which patient subgroups will benefit more or less from ICD therapy than that demonstrated in the above referenced publication. . . . Whether the recommendation to implant ICDs in post-myocardial infarction patients with LV ejection fraction of 30% or less should be limited to individuals these high-risk variables awaits further clarification . . . "

In reality, in many countries economic considerations determine the level of healthcare achieved. The gap between what is medically possible and the resources available is increasing rapidly. It appears judicious to adapt the guidelines to take socioeconomic considerations into account. However, this would be contrary to the intention of the guidelines, since their purpose is to recommend what can be considered to be the best evidence-based management strategy in a particular situation. It is the responsibility of healthcare authorities to put guidelines in the economic context of a specific health care system and to decide which therapies will be reimbursed.[4]

Medicine is an art that has to take individual patients' needs into account, even in the presence of guidelines.[165] Therefore, indiscriminate application of guidelines to each and every patient does not automatically constitute a guarantee of good clinical practice (Table 5).

References

1. Mirowski M, Reid PR, Mower MM, Watkins L, Gott VL, Schauble JF, Langer A, Heilman MS, Kolenik S, Fischell RE, Weisfeldt M. Termination of malignant ventricular arrhythmias with an implanted automatic defibrillator in human beings. N Engl J Med 1980;303:322–324.
2. Moss AJ, Hall WJ, Cannom DS, Daubert JP, Higgins SL, Klein H, Levine JH, Saksena S, Waldo AL, Wilber D,

Brown MW, Heo M, MADIT Investigators. Improved survival with an implanted defibrillator in patients with coronary disease at high risk for ventricular arrhythmia. N Engl J Med 1996;335:1933–1940.

3. Fogoros RN. Impact of the implantable defibrillator on mortality: the axiom of overall implantable cardioverter-defibrillator survival. Am J Cardiol 1996; 78:57–61.

4. Priori SG, Klein W, Bassand JP. Medical Practice Guidelines. Separating science from economics. Eur Heart J 2003;24:1962–1964.

5. Dreifus LS, Fisch C, Griffin JC, Gillette PC, Mason JW, Parsonnet V. Guidelines for implantation of cardiac pacemakers and antiarrhythmia devices. A report of the American College of Cardiology/American Heart Association Task Force on Assessment of Diagnostic and Therapeutic Cardiovascular Procedures. (Committee on Pacemaker Implantation). Circulation 1991;84:455–467.

6. Gregoratos G, Cheitlin MD, Conill A, Epstein AE, Fellows C, Ferguson TBJ, Freedman RA, Hlatky MA, Naccarelli GV, Saksena S, Schlant RC, Silka MJ. ACC/AHA Guidelines for Implantation of Cardiac Pacemakers and Antiarrhythmia Devices: Executive Summary–a report of the American College of Cardiology/American Heart Association Task Force on Practice Guidelines (Committee on Pacemaker Implantation). Circulation 1998;97:1325–1335.

7. Gregoratos G, Abrams J, Epstein AE, Freedman RA, Hayes DL, Hlatky MA, Kerber RE, Naccarelli GV, Schoenfeld MH, Silka MJ, Winters SL. ACC/AHA/ NASPE 2002 Guideline Update for Implantation of Cardiac Pacemakers and Antiarrhythmia Devices– summary article: a report of the American College of

Cardiology/American Heart Association Task Force on Practice Guidelines (ACC/AHA/NASPE Committee to Update the 1998 Pacemaker Guidelines). J Am Coll Cardiol 2002;40:1703–1719.

8. Working Groups on Cardiac Arrhythmias and Cardiac Pacing of the European Society of Cardiology. Guidelines for the use of implantable cardioverter defibrillators. A Task Force of the Working Groups on Cardiac Arrhythmias and Cardiac Pacing of the European Society of Cardiology. Eur Heart J 1992;13:1304–1310.

9. Hauer RN, Aliot E, Block M, Capucci A, Luderitz B, Santini M, Vardas PE. Indications for implantable cardioverter defibrillator (ICD) therapy. Study Group on Guidelines on ICDs of the Working Group on Arrhythmias and the Working Group on Cardiac Pacing of the European Society of Cardiology. Eur Heart J 2001;22:1074–1081.

10. Priori SG, Aliot E, Blomstrom-Lundqvist C, Bossaert L, Breithardt G, Brugada P, Camm JA, Cappato R, Cobbe SM, Di Mario C, Maron BJ, McKenna WJ, Pedersen AK, Ravens U, Schwartz PJ, Trusz-Gluza M, Vardas P, Wellens HJ, Zipes DP. Update of the guidelines on sudden cardiac death of the European Society of Cardiology. Eur Heart J 2003;24:13–15.

11. Steinbeck G. Evolution of implantable cardioverter defibrillator indications: comparison of guidelines in the United States and Europe. J Cardiovasc Electrophysiol 2002;13:S96–S99.

12. Gregoratos G, Cheitlin MD, Conill A, Epstein AE, Fellows C, Ferguson TBJ, Freedman RA, Hlatky MA, Naccarelli GV, Saksena S, Schlant RC, Silka MJ, Ritchie JL, Gibbons RJ, Eagle KA, Gardner TJ, Lewis RP, O'Rourke RA, Ryan TJ, Garson A, Jr. ACC/AHA guidelines for implantation of cardiac pacemakers and

antiarrhythmia devices: a report of the American College of Cardiology/American Heart Association Task Force on Practice Guidelines (Committee on Pacemaker Implantation). J Am Coll Cardiol 1998;31:1175–1209.

13. Luu M, Stevenson WG, Stevenson LW, Baron K, Walden J. Diverse mechanisms of unexpected cardiac arrest in advanced heart failure. Circulation 1989;80:1675–1680.

14. Bayes de Luna A, Coumel P, Leclercq JF. Ambulatory sudden cardiac death: mechanisms of production of fatal arrhythmia on the basis of data from 157 cases. Am Heart J 1989;117:151–159.

15. Saksena S, Poczobutt Johanos M, Castle LW, Fogoros RN, Alpert BL, Kron J, Pacifico A, Griffin J, Ruskin JN, Kehoe RF, Yee R, Dorian P, Kerr CR, Luceri RM, Poliseno M. Long-term multicenter experience with a second-generation implantable pacemaker-defibrillator in patients with malignant ventricular tachyarrhythmias. J Am Coll Cardiol 1992;19:490–499.

16. Bardy GH, Troutman C, Poole JE, Kudenchuk PJ, Dolack GL, Johnson G, Hofer B. Clinical experience with a tiered-therapy, multiprogrammable antiarrhythmia device. Circulation 1992;85:1689–1698.

17. Winkle RA, Mead RH, Ruder MA, Gaudiani VA, Smith NA, Buch WS, Schmidt P, Shipman T. Long-term outcome with the automatic implantable cardioverter-defibrillator. J Am Coll Cardiol 1989;13:1353–1361.

18. Fogoros RN, Elson JJ, Bonnet CA, Fiedler SB, Burkholder JA. Efficacy of the automatic implantable cardioverter-defibrillator in prolonging survival in patients with severe underlying cardiac disease. J Am Coll Cardiol 1990;16:381–386.

19. Böcker D, Block M, Isbruch F, Wietholt D, Hammel D, Borggrefe M, Breithardt G. Do patients with an implantable defibrillator live longer? J Am Coll Cardiol 1993;21:1638–1644.
20. Böcker D, Block M, Isbruch F, Fastenrath C, Castrucci M, Hammel D, Scheld HH, Borggrefe M, Breithardt G. Benefits of treatment with implantable cardioverter-defibrillators in patients with stable ventricular tachycardia without cardiac arrest. Br Heart J 1995;73: 158–163.
21. Böcker D, Bänsch D, Heinecke A, Weber M, Brunn J, Hammel D, Borggrefe M, Breithardt G, Block M. Potential benefit from implantable cardioverter-defibrillator therapy in patients with and without heart failure. Circulation 1998;98:1636–1643.
22. Kim SG. Implantable defibrillator therapy: Does it really prolong life? How can we prove it? Am J Cardiol 1993;71:1213–1218.
23. Kuck KH, Cappato R, Siebels J, Ruppel R. Randomized comparison of antiarrhythmic drug therapy with implantable defibrillators in patients resuscitated from cardiac arrest: The Cardiac Arrest Study Hamburg (CASH). Circulation 2000;102:748–754.
24. Connolly SJ, Gent M, Roberts RS, Dorian P, Roy D, Sheldon RS, Mitchell LB, Green MS, Klein GJ, O'Brien B. Canadian Implantable Defibrillator Study (CIDS): A randomized trial of the implantable cardioverter defibrillator against amiodarone. Circulation 2000;101:1297–1302.
25. The Antiarrhythmics versus Implantable Defibrillators (AVID) Investigators. A comparison of antiarrhythmic-drug therapy with implantable defibrillators in patients resuscitated from near-fatal ventricular arrhythmias. N Engl J Med 1997;337:1576–1583.

26. Brouwer IA, Zock PL, Wever EF, Hauer RN, Camm AJ, Böcker D, Otto-Terlouw P, Katan MB, Schouten EG. Rationale and design of a randomised controlled clinical trial on supplemental intake of n-3 fatty acids and incidence of cardiac arrhythmia: SOFA. Eur J Clin Nutr 2003;57:1323–1330.
27. Steinbeck G, Andresen D, Bach P, Haberl R, Oeff M, Hoffmann E, Von Leitner ER. A comparison of electrophysiologically guided antiarrhythmic drug therapy with beta-blocker therapy in patients with symptomatic, sustained ventricular tachyarrhythmias. N Engl J Med 1992;
28. Cardiac Arrhythmia Suppression Trial (CAST) Investigators. Effect of antiarrhythmic agent moricizine on survival after myocardial infarction. N Engl J Med 1992;327:227–233.
29. Cardiac Arrhythmia Suppression Trial (CAST) Investigators. Effect of encainide and flecainide on mortality in infarction. N Engl J Med 1989;321:406–412.
30. Belhassen B, Viskin S, Fish R, Glick A, Setbon I, Eldar M. Effects of electrophysiologic-guided therapy with Class IA antiarrhythmic drugs on the long-term outcome of patients with idiopathic ventricular fibrillation with or without the Brugada syndrome. J Cardiovasc Electrophysiol 1999;10:1301–1312.
31. Cairns JA, Connolly SJ, Roberts R, Gent M, the Canadian Amiodarone Myocardial Infarction Arrhythmia Trial Investigators. Randomised trial of outcome after myocardial infarction in patients with frequent or repetitive ventricular premature depolarisations: CAMIAT. Lancet 1997;349:675–682.
32. Julian DG, Camm AJ, Frangin G, Janse MJ, Munoz A, Schwartz PJ, Simon P, the European Myocardial Infarct Amiodarone Trial Investigators. Randomised trial of effect of amiodarone on mortality in patients

with left-ventricular dysfunction after recent myocardial infarction: EMIAT. Lancet 1997;349:667–674.

33. Boutitie F, Boissel JP, Connolly SJ, Camm AJ, Cairns JA, Julian DG, Gent M, Janse MJ, Dorian P, Frangin G. Amiodarone interaction with beta-blockers: Analysis of the merged EMIAT (European Myocardial Infarct Amiodarone Trial) and CAMIAT (Canadian Amiodarone Myocardial Infarction Trial) databases. The EMIAT and CAMIAT Investigators. Circulation 1999;99:2268–2275.

34. Strickberger SA, Man KC, Daoud E, Goyal R, Brinkman K, Hasse C, Bogun F, Knight BP, Weiss R, Bahu M, Morady F. A prospective evaluation of catheter ablation of ventricular tachycardia as adjuvant therapy in patients with coronary artery disease and an implatable cardioverter-defibrillator. Circulation 1997;96:1525–1531.

35. Haissaguerre M, Extramiana F, Hocini M, Cauchemez B, Jais P, Cabrera JA, Farre G, Leenhardt A, Sanders P, Scavee C, Hsu LF, Weerasooriya R, Shah DC, Frank R, Maury P, Delay M, Garrigue S, Clementy J. Mapping and ablation of ventricular fibrillation associated with long-QT and Brugada syndromes. Circulation 2003;108:925–928.

36. Kottkamp H, Wetzel U, Schirdewahn P, Dorszewski A, Gerds-Li JH, Carbucicchio C, Kobza R, Hindricks G. Catheter ablation of ventricular tachycardia in remote myocardial infarction: Substrate description guiding placement of individual linear lesions targeting noninducibility. J Cardiovasc Electrophysiol 2003;14:675–681.

37. Klein LS, Shih HT, Hackett FK, Zipes DP, Miles WM. Radiofrequency catheter ablation of ventricular

tachycardia in patients without structural heart disease. Circulation 1992;85:1666–1674.

38. Böcker D, Haverkamp W, Block M, Hammel D, Borggrefe M, Breithardt G. Comparison of d,l-sotalol and implantable defibrillators for treatment of sustained ventricular tachycardia or fibrillation in patients with coronary artery disease. Circulation 1996;94:151–157.

39. Newman D, Sauve MJ, Herre J, Langberg JJ, Lee MA, Titus C, Franklin J, Scheinman MM, Griffin JC. Survival after implantation of the cardioverter defibrillator. Am J Cardiol 1992;69:899–903.

40. Strickberger SA, Hummel JD, Bartlett TG, Frumin HI, Schuger CD, Beau SL, Bitar C, Morady F. Amiodarone versus implantable cardioverter-defibrillator: randomized trial in patients with nonischemic dilated cardiomyopathy and asymptomatic nonsustained ventricular tachycardia—AMIOVIRT. J Am Coll Cardiol 2003;41:1707–1712.

41. Wever EF, Hauer RNW, Van Capelle FJL, Tijssen JGP, Crijns HJGM, Algra A, Wiesfeld ACP, Bakker PFA, Robles de Medina EO. Randomized study of implantable defibrillator as first-choice therapy versus conventional postinfarct sudden death survivors. Circulation 1995;91:2195–2203.

42. Moss AJ, Zareba W, Hall WJ, Klein H, Wilber DJ, Cannom DS, Daubert JP, Higgins SL, Brown MW, Andrews ML. Prophylactic implantation of a defibrillator in patients with myocardial infarction and reduced ejection fraction. N Engl J Med 2002;346:877–883.

43. Bänsch D, Antz M, Boczor S, Volkmer M, Tebbenjohanns J, Seidl K, Block M, Gietzen F, Berger J, Kuck KH. Primary prevention of sudden cardiac death in

idiopathic dilated cardiomyopathy: the Cardiomyopathy Trial (CAT). Circulation 2002;105:1453–1458.
44. Nademanee K, Veerakul G, Mower M, Likittanasombat K, Krittayapong R, Bhuripanyo K, Sitthisook S, Chaothawee L, Lai MY, Azen SP. Defibrillator versus beta-blockers for unexplained death in Thailand (debut): A randomized clinical trial. Circulation 2003;107:2221–2226.
45. Nisam S, Mower M. ICD trials: An extraordinary means of determining patient risk? Pacing Clin Electrophysiol 1998;21:1341–1346.
46. Bigger JT, Jr., Coronary Artery Bypass Graft (CABG) Patch Trial Investigators. Prophylactic use of implanted cardiac defibrillators in patients at high risk for ventricular arrhythmias after coronary-artery bypass graft surgery. New England J Med 1997;337: 1569–1575.
47. Buxton AE, Lee KL, Fisher JD, Josephson ME, Prystowsky EN, Hafley G. A randomized study of the prevention of sudden death in patients with coronary artery disease. Multicenter Unsustained Tachycardia Trial Investigators. N Engl J Med 1999;341:1882–1890.
48. Hohnloser SH, Connolly SJ, Kuck KH, Dorian P, Fain E, Hampton JR, Hatala R, Pauly AC, Roberts RS, Themeles E, Gent M. The defibrillator in acute myocardial infarction trial (DINAMIT): study protocol. Am Heart J 2000;140:735–739.
49. Breithardt G, Cain ME, El Sherif N, Flowers N, Hombach V, Janse M, Simson MB, Steinbeck G. Standards for analysis of ventricular late potentials using high resolution or signal-averaged electrocardiography. A statement by a Task Force Committee between the European Society of Cardiology, the American

Heart Association and the American College of Cardiology. Eur Heart J 1991;12:473–480.

50. Böcker D, Shenasa M, Borggrefe M, Fetsch T, Breithardt G. Late potentials, heart rate variability, and electrocardiography. Curr Opin Cardiol 1993;8:39–53.

51. Breithardt G, Borggrefe M, Fetsch T, Böcker D, Mäkijärvi M, Reinhardt L, Mäkijärvi M. Prognosis and risk stratification after myocardial infarction. Eur Heart J 1995;16:10–19.

52. Bigger JT, Jr., Whang W, Rottman JN, Kleiger RE, Gottlieb CD, Namerow PB, Steinman RC, Estes NA. Mechanisms of death in the CABG Patch trial: A randomized trial of implantable cardiac defibrillator prophylaxis in patients at high risk of death after coronary artery bypass graft surgery. Circulation 1999;99: 1416–1421.

53. Kleiger RE, Miller JP, Bigger JT, Jr., Moss AJ, The Multicenter Post-Infarction Research Group. Decreased heart rate variability and its association with increased mortality after myocardial infarction. Am J Cardiol 1987;59:256–262.

54. La Rovere MT, Bigger JT, Jr., Marcus FI, Mortara A, Schwartz PJ, ATRAMI (Autonomic Tone and Reflexes After Myocardial Infarction) Investigators. Baroreflex sensitivity and heart-rate variability in prediction of total cardiac mortality after myocardial infarction. Lancet 1998;351:478–484.

55. Gruberg L. DINAMIT: The Defibrillator in Acute Myocardial Infarction Trial. Internet communication, accessed at: http://www.medscape.com/viewarticle/ 472003 on 3/25/2004.

56. Davies LC, Francis DP, Ponikowski P, Piepoli MF, Coats AJ. Relation of heart rate and blood pressure turbulence following premature ventricular complexes to

baroreflex sensitivity in chronic congestive heart failure. Am J Cardiol 2001;87:737–742.

57. Lin LY, Lai LP, Lin JL, Du CC, Shau WY, Chan HL, Tseng YZ, Huang SK. Tight mechanism correlation between heart rate turbulence and baroreflex sensitivity: sequential autonomic blockade analysis. J Cardiovasc Electrophysiol 2002;13:427–431.

58. Wichterle D, Melenovsky V, Malik M. Mechanisms involved in heart rate turbulence. Card Electrophysiol Rev 2002;6:262–266.

59. Schmidt G, Malik M, Barthel P, Schneider R, Ulm K, Rolnitzky L, Camm AJ, Bigger JT, Jr., Schomig A. Heart-rate turbulence after ventricular premature beats as a predictor of mortality after acute myocardial infarction. Lancet 1999;353:1390–1396.

60. Ghuran A, Reid F, La Rovere MT, Schmidt G, Bigger JT, Jr., Camm AJ, Schwartz PJ, Malik M. Heart rate turbulence-based predictors of fatal and nonfatal cardiac arrest (The Autonomic Tone and Reflexes After Myocardial Infarction substudy). Am J Cardiol 2002;89:184–190.

61. Barthel P, Schneider R, Bauer A, Ulm K, Schmitt C, Schomig A, Schmidt G. Risk stratification after acute myocardial infarction by heart rate turbulence. Circulation 2003;108:1221–1226.

62. Hohnloser SH, Klingenheben T, Li YG, Zabel M, Peetermans J, Cohen RJ. T wave alternans as a predictor of recurrent ventricular tachyarrhythmias in ICD recipients: prospective comparison with conventional risk markers. J Cardiovasc Electrophysiol 1998;9:1258–1268.

63. Tapanainen JM, Still AM, Airaksinen KE, Huikuri HV. Prognostic significance of risk stratifiers of mortality, including T wave alternans, after acute myocardial

infarction: results of a prospective follow-up study. J Cardiovasc Electrophysiol 2001;12:645–652.

64. Ikeda T, Sakata T, Takami M, Kondo N, Tezuka N, Nakae T, Noro M, Enjoji Y, Abe R, Sugi K, Yamaguchi T. Combined assessment of T-wave alternans and late potentials used to predict arrhythmic events after myocardial infarction. A prospective study. J Am Coll Cardiol 2000;35:722–730.

65. Wever EF, Hauer RN, Schrijvers G, van Capelle FJ, Tijssen JG, Crijns HJ, Algra A, Ramanna H, Bakker PF, Robles de Medina EO. Cost-effectiveness of implantable defibrillator as first-choice therapy versus electrophysiologically guided, tiered strategy in postinfarct sudden death survivors. A randomized study. Circulation 1996;93:489–496.

66. Connolly SJ, Gent M, Roberts RS, Dorian P, Green MS, Klein GJ, Mitchell LB, Sheldon RS, Roy D. Canadian implantable defibrillator study (CIDS): Study design and organization. Am J Cardiol 1993;72:103F–108F.

67. Siebels J, Kuck KH. Implantable cardioverter defibrillator compared with antiarrhythmic drug treatment in cardiac arrest survivors (the Cardiac Arrest Study Hamburg). Am Heart J 1994;127:1139–1144.

68. Connolly SJ, Hallstrom AP, Cappato R, Schron EB, Kuck KH, Zipes DP, Greene HL, Boczor S, Domanski M, Follmann D, Gent M, Roberts RS. Meta-analysis of the implantable cardioverter defibrillator secondary prevention trials. AVID, CASH and CIDS studies. Antiarrhythmics vs Implantable Defibrillator study. Cardiac Arrest Study Hamburg. Canadian Implantable Defibrillator Study. Eur Heart J 2000;21:2071–2078.

69. Sheldon R, Connolly S, Krahn A, Roberts R, Gent M, Gardner M. Identification of patients most likely

to benefit from implantable cardioverter-defibrillator therapy: The Canadian Implantable Defibrillator Study [see comments]. Circulation 2000;101:1660–1664.

70. Sheldon R, O'Brien BJ, Blackhouse G, Goeree R, Mitchell B, Klein G, Roberts RS, Gent M, Connolly SJ. Effect of clinical risk stratification on cost-effectiveness of the implantable cardioverter-defibrillator: The Canadian implantable defibrillator study. Circulation 2001;104:1622–1626.

71. Anderson JL, Hallstrom AP, Epstein AE, Pinski SL, Rosenberg Y, Nora MO, Chilson DA, Cannom DS, Moore R, The Antiarrhythmics versus Implantable Defibrillators (AVID) Investigators. Design and results of the antiarrhythmics vs implantable defibrillators (AVID) registry. Circulation 1999;99:1692–1699.

72. Reynolds MR, Josephson ME. MADIT II (second Multicenter Automated Defibrillator Implantation Trial) debate: risk stratification, costs, and public policy. Circulation 2003;108:1779–1783.

73. Plummer CJ, Irving RJ, McComb JM. Implications of national guidance for implantable cardioverter defibrillation implantation in the United Kingdom. Pacing Clin Electrophysiol 2003;26:479–482.

74. Moss AJ. Implantable cardioverter defibrillator therapy: the sickest patients benefit the most. Circulation 2000;101:1638–1640.

75. Moss AJ, Fadl Y, Zareba W, Cannom DS, Hall WJ. Survival benefit with an implanted defibrillator in relation to mortality risk in chronic coronary heart disease. Am J Cardiol 2001;88:516–520.

76. Gomes JA, Cain ME, Buxton AE, Josephson ME, Lee KL, Hafley GE. Prediction of long-term outcomes by signal-averaged electrocardiography in patients with

unsustained ventricular tachycardia, coronary artery disease, and left ventricular dysfunction. Circulation 2001;104:436–441.

77. Zareba, W. Noninvasive Electrocardiology and Outcome in MADIT II Patients. Internet communication, accessed at: http://www.madit2.com/issue3/ issue3_en/articles/zareba.htm on 12/25/2003.

78. Bardy GH. SCD-HeFT: The Sudden Cardiac Death in Heart Failure Trial. Internet communication, accessed at: http://www.sicr.org/scdheft_results_acc_lbcc.pdf on 3/25/2004.

79. Knight BP, Goyal R, Pelosi F, Flemming M, Horwood L, Morady F, Strickberger SA. Outcome of patients with nonischemic dilated cardiomyopathy and unexplained syncope treated with an implantable defibrillator. J Am Coll Cardiol 1999;33:1964–1970.

80. Fonarow GC, Feliciano Z, Boyle NG, Knight L, Woo MA, Moriguchi JD, Laks H, Wiener I. Improved survival in patients with nonischemic advanced heart failure and syncope treated with an implantable cardioverter-defibrillator. Am J Cardiol 2000;85:981–985.

81. Bänsch D, Böcker D, Brunn J, Weber M, Breithardt G, Block M. Clusters of ventricular tachycardias signify impaired survival in patients with idiopathic dilated cardiomyopathy and implantable cardioverter defibrillators. J Am Coll Cardiol 2000;36:566–573.

82. Kadish A, Quigg R, Schaechter A, Anderson KP, Estes M, Levine J. Defibrillators in nonischemic cardiomyopathy treatment evaluation. Pacing Clin Electrophysiol 2000;23:338–343.

83. Kadish, A. H. Defibrillators in nonischemic cardiomyopathy treatment evaluation [DEFINITE]. Internet communication, accessed at: http://www.medscape .com/viewarticle/464980 on 12/25/2003.

84. Massie BM, Fisher SG, Deedwania PC, Singh BN, Fletcher RD, Singh SN. Effect of amiodarone on clinical status and left ventricular function in patients with congestive heart failure. CHF-STAT Investigators. Circulation 1996;93:2128–2134.

85. Grimm W, Christ M, Bach J, Muller HH, Maisch B. Noninvasive arrhythmia risk stratification in idiopathic dilated cardiomyopathy: Results of the Marburg Cardiomyopathy Study. Circulation 2003;108: 2883–2891.

86. Hohnloser SH, Klingenheben T, Bloomfield D, Dabbous O, Cohen RJ. Usefulness of microvolt T-wave alternans for prediction of ventricular tachyarrhythmic events in patients with dilated cardiomyopathy: Results from a prospective observational study. J Am Coll Cardiol 2003;41:2220–2224.

87. Brugada P, Brugada J. Right bundle branch block, persistent ST segment elevation and sudden cardiac death: A distinct clinical and electrocardiographic syndrome. A multicenter report. J Am Coll Cardiol 1992;20:1391–1396.

88. Wilde AA, Antzelevitch C, Borggrefe M, Brugada J, Brugada R, Brugada P, Corrado D, Hauer RN, Kass RS, Nademanee K, Priori SG, Towbin JA. Proposed diagnostic criteria for the Brugada syndrome. Eur Heart J 2002;23:1648–1654.

89. Brugada R, Brugada J, Antzelevitch C, Kirsch GE, Potenza D, Towbin JA, Brugada P. Sodium channel blockers identify risk for sudden death in patients with ST-segment elevation and right bundle branch block but structurally normal hearts. Circulation 2000;101:510–515.

90. Rolf S, Bruns HJ, Wichter T, Kirchhof P, Ribbing M, Wasmer K, Paul M, Breithardt G, Haverkamp W, Eckardt L. The ajmaline challenge in Brugada

syndrome: diagnostic impact, safety, and recommended protocol. Eur Heart J 2003;24:1104–1112.

91. Miyazaki T, Mitamura H, Miyoshi S, Soejima K, Aizawa Y, Ogawa S. Autonomic and antiarrhythmic drug modulation of ST segment elevation in patients with Brugada syndrome. J Am Coll Cardiol 1996;27:1061–1070.

92. Dumaine R, Towbin JA, Brugada P, Vatta M, Nesterenko DV, Nesterenko VV, Brugada J, Brugada R, Antzelevitch C. Ionic mechanisms responsible for the electrocardiographic phenotype of the Brugada syndrome are temperature dependent [see comments]. Circ Res 1999;85:803–809.

93. Gussak I, Antzelevitch C. Early repolarization syndrome: clinical characteristics and possible cellular and ionic mechanisms. J Electrocardiol 2000;33:299–309.

94. Vatta M, Dumaine R, Varghese G, Richard TA, Shimizu W, Aihara N, Nademanee K, Brugada R, Brugada J, Veerakul G, Li H, Bowles NE, Brugada P, Antzelevitch C, Towbin JA. Genetic and biophysical basis of sudden unexplained nocturnal death syndrome (SUNDS), a disease allelic to Brugada syndrome. Hum Mol Genet 2002;11:337–345.

95. Yan GX, Antzelevitch C. Cellular basis for the Brugada syndrome and other mechanisms of arrhythmogenesis associated with ST-segment elevation. Circulation 1999;100:1660–1666.

96. Brugada J, Brugada R, Brugada P. Determinants of sudden cardiac death in individuals with the electrocardiographic pattern of Brugada syndrome and no previous cardiac arrest. Circulation 2003;108:3092–6.

97. Gasparini M, Priori SG, Mantica M, Coltorti F, Napolitano C, Galimberti P, Bloise R, Ceriotti C. Programmed electrical stimulation in Brugada syndrome:

How reproducible are the results? J Cardiovasc Electrophysiol 2002;13:880–887.

98. Eckardt L, Kirchhof P, Schulze-Bahr E, Rolf S, Ribbing M, Loh P, Bruns HJ, Witte A, Milberg P, Borggrefe M, Breithardt G, Wichter T, Haverkamp W. Electrophysiologic investigation in Brugada syndrome: Yield of programmed ventricular stimulation at two ventricular sites with up to three premature beats. Eur Heart J 2002;23:1394–1401.

99. Priori SG, Napolitano C, Gasparini M, Pappone C, Della BP, Giordano U, Bloise R, Giustetto C, De Nardis R, Grillo M, Ronchetti E, Faggiano G, Nastoli J. Natural history of Brugada syndrome: Insights for risk stratification and management. Circulation 2002;105:1342–1347.

100. Antzelevitch C. Molecular genetics of arrhythmias and cardiovascular conditions associated with arrhythmias. Pacing Clin Electrophysiol 2003;26: 2194–2208.

101. Geier C, Perrot A, Ozcelik C, Binner P, Counsell D, Hoffmann K, Pilz B, Martiniak Y, Gehmlich K, van der Ven PF, Furst DO, Vornwald A, von Hodenberg E, Nurnberg P, Scheffold T, Dietz R, Osterziel KJ. Mutations in the human muscle LIM protein gene in families with hypertrophic cardiomyopathy. Circulation 2003;107:1390–1395.

102. Watkins H. Genetic clues to disease pathways in hypertrophic and dilated cardiomyopathies. Circulation 2003;107:1344–1346.

103. Marian AJ, Salek L, Lutucuta S. Molecular genetics and pathogenesis of hypertrophic cardiomyopathy. Minerva Med 2001;92:435–451.

104. McKenna WJ, Behr ER. Hypertrophic cardiomyopathy: management, risk stratification, and prevention of sudden death. Heart 2002;87:169–176.

105. Maron BJ, McKenna WJ, Danielson GK, Kappenberger LJ, Kuhn HJ, Seidman CE, Shah PM, Spencer WH, III, Spirito P, ten Cate FJ, Wigle ED, Vogel RA, Abrams J, Bates ER, Brodie BR, Danias PG, Gregoratos G, Hlatky MA, Hochman JS, Kaul S, Lichtenberg RC, Lindner JR, O'Rourke RA, Pohost GM, Schofield RS, Tracy CM, Winters WL, Jr., Klein WW, Priori SG, Alonso-Garcia A, Blomstrom-Lundqvist C, De Backer G, Deckers J, Flather M, Hradec J, Oto A, Parkhomenko A, Silber S, Torbicki A. American College of Cardiology/European Society of Cardiology Clinical Expert Consensus Document on Hypertrophic Cardiomyopathy. A report of the American College of Cardiology Foundation Task Force on Clinical Expert Consensus Documents and the European Society of Cardiology Committee for Practice Guidelines. Eur Heart J 2003;24:1965–1991.

106. McKenna WJ, Oakley CM, Krikler DM, Goodwin JF. Improved survival with amiodarone in patients with hypertrophic cardiomyopathy and ventricular tachycardia. Br Heart J 1985;53:412–416.

107. Elliott PM, Sharma S, Varnava A, Poloniecki J, Rowland E, McKenna WJ. Survival after cardiac arrest or sustained ventricular tachycardia in patients with hypertrophic cardiomyopathy. J Am Coll Cardiol 1999;33:1596–1601.

108. Maron BJ, Shen WK, Link MS, Epstein AE, Almquist AK, Daubert JP, Bardy GH, Favale S, Rea RF, Boriani G, Estes NA, III, Spirito P. Efficacy of implantable cardioverter-defibrillators for the prevention of sudden death in patients with hypertrophic cardiomyopathy. N Engl J Med 2000;342:365–373.

109. Monserrat L, Elliott PM, Gimeno JR, Sharma S, Penas-Lado M, McKenna WJ. Non-sustained ventricular tachycardia in hypertrophic cardiomyopathy:

An independent marker of sudden death risk in young patients. J Am Coll Cardiol 2003;42:873–879.

110. Hess OM. Risk stratification in hypertrophic cardiomyopathy: Fact or fiction? J Am Coll Cardiol 2003;42:880–881.

111. Elliott PM, Poloniecki J, Dickie S, Sharma S, Monserrat L, Varnava A, Mahon NG, McKenna WJ. Sudden death in hypertrophic cardiomyopathy: identification of high risk patients. J Am Coll Cardiol 2000;36:2212–2218.

112. Elliott PM, Gimeno B, Jr., Mahon NG, Poloniecki JD, McKenna WJ. Relation between severity of left-ventricular hypertrophy and prognosis in patients with hypertrophic cardiomyopathy. Lancet 2001; 357:420–424.

113. Maron BJ, Piccininno M, Casey SA, Bernabo P, Spirito P. Relation of extreme left ventricular hypertrophy to age in hypertrophic cardiomyopathy. Am J Cardiol 2003;91:626–628.

114. Ackerman MJ, VanDriest SL, Ommen SR, Will ML, Nishimura RA, Tajik AJ, Gersh BJ. Prevalence and age-dependence of malignant mutations in the beta-myosin heavy chain and troponin T genes in hypertrophic cardiomyopathy: A comprehensive outpatient perspective. J Am Coll Cardiol 2002;39: 2042–2048.

115. Van Driest SL, Ackerman MJ, Ommen SR, Shakur R, Will ML, Nishimura RA, Tajik AJ, Gersh BJ. Prevalence and severity of "benign" mutations in the beta-myosin heavy chain, cardiac troponin T, and alpha-tropomyosin genes in hypertrophic cardiomyopathy. Circulation 2002;106:3085–3090.

116. Woo A, Rakowski H, Liew JC, Zhao MS, Liew CC, Parker TG, Zeller M, Wigle ED, Sole MJ. Mutations

of the beta myosin heavy chain gene in hypertrophic cardiomyopathy: Critical functional sites determine prognosis. Heart 2003;89:1179–1185.

117. Van Driest SL, Maron BJ, Ackerman MJ. From malignant mutations to malignant domains: The continuing search for prognostic significance in the mutant genes causing hypertrophic cardiomyopathy. Heart 2004;90:7–8.

118. Cecchi F, Olivotto I, Montereggi A, Squillatini G, Dolara A, Maron BJ. Prognostic value of non-sustained ventricular tachycardia and the potential role of amiodarone treatment in hypertrophic cardiomyopathy: Assessment in an unselected non-referral based patient population [see comments]. Heart 1998;79:331–336.

119. Moss AJ, Schwartz PJ, Crampton RS, Locati E, Carleen E. The long QT syndrome: A prospective international study. Circulation 1985;71:17–21.

120. Moss AJ, Schwartz PJ, Crampton RS, Tzivoni D, Locati EH, MacCluer J, Hall WJ, Weitkamp L, Vincent GM, Garson A, Jr. The long QT syndrome. Prospective longitudinal study of 328 families. Circulation 1991;84:1136–1144.

121. Schwartz PJ, Locati E. The idiopathic long QT syndrome: Pathogenetic mechanisms and therapy. Eur Heart J 1985;6 (Suppl D):103–114.

122. Camm AJ, Janse MJ, Roden DM, Rosen MR, Cinca J, Cobbe SM. Congenital and acquired long QT syndrome. Eur Heart J 2000;21:1232–1237.

123. Zareba W, Moss AJ, Locati EH, Lehmann MH, Peterson DR, Hall WJ, Schwartz PJ, Vincent GM, Priori SG, Benhorin J, Towbin JA, Robinson JL, Andrews ML, Napolitano C, Timothy K, Zhang L, Medina A. Modulating effects of age and gender

on the clinical course of long QT syndrome by genotype. J Am Coll Cardiol 2003;42:103–109.

124. Priori SG, Schwartz PJ, Napolitano C, Bloise R, Ronchetti E, Grillo M, Vicentini A, Spazzolini C, Nastoli J, Bottelli G, Folli R, Cappelletti D. Risk stratification in the long-QT syndrome. N Engl J Med 2003;348:1866–1874.

125. Priori SG, Aliot E, Blomstrom-Lundqvist C, Bossaert L, Breithardt G, Brugada P, Camm JA, Cappato R, Cobbe SM, Di MC, Maron BJ, McKenna WJ, Pedersen AK, Ravens U, Schwartz PJ, Trusz-Gluza M, Vardas P, Wellens HJ, Zipes DP. Task Force on sudden cardiac death, European Society of Cardiology. Europace 2002;4:3–18.

126. Chiang CE, Roden DM. The long QT syndromes: Genetic basis and clinical implications. J Am Coll Cardiol 2000;36:1–12.

127. Zareba W, Moss AJ, Daubert JP, Hall WJ, Robinson JL, Andrews M. Implantable cardioverter defibrillator in high-risk long QT syndrome patients. J Cardiovasc Electrophysiol 2003;14:337–341.

128. Viskin S. Implantable cardioverter defibrillator in high-risk long QT syndrome patients. J Cardiovasc Electrophysiol 2003;14:1130–1131.

129. Gussak I, Brugada P, Brugada J, Wright RS, Kopecky SL, Chaitman BR, Bjerregaard P. Idiopathic short QT interval: A new clinical syndrome? Cardiology 2000;94:99–102.

130. Gaita F, Giustetto C, Bianchi F, Wolpert C, Schimpf R, Riccardi R, Grossi S, Richiardi E, Borggrefe M. Short QT Syndrome: A familial cause of sudden death. Circulation 2003;108:965–970.

131. Brugada R, Hong K, Dumaine R, Cordeiro J, Gaita F, Borggrefe M, Menendez TM, Brugada J, Pollevick

GD, Wolpert C, Burashnikov E, Matsuo K, Sheng WY, Guerchicoff A, Bianchi F, Giustetto C, Schimpf R, Brugada P, Antzelevitch C. Sudden death associated with short-qt syndrome linked to mutations in HERG. Circulation 2003;108:3092–6.

132. Schimpf R, Wolpert C, Bianchi F, Giustetto C, Gaita F, Bauersfeld U, Borggrefe M. Congenital short QT syndrome and implantable cardioverter defibrillator treatment: inherent risk for inappropriate shock delivery. J Cardiovasc Electrophysiol 2003;14:1273–1277.

133. Marcus FI, Fontaine GH, Guiraudon G, Frank R, Laurenceau JL, Malergue C, Grosgogeat Y. Right ventricular dysplasia: A report of 24 adult cases. Circulation 1982;65:384–398.

134. Tabib A, Loire R, Chalabreysse L, Meyronnet D, Miras A, Malicier D, Thivolet F, Chevalier P, Bouvagnet P. Circumstances of death and gross and microscopic observations in a series of 200 cases of sudden death associated with arrhythmogenic right ventricular cardiomyopathy and/or dysplasia. Circulation 2003;108:3000–3005.

135. Tiso N, Stephan DA, Nava A, Bagattin A, Devaney JM, Stanchi F, Larderet G, Brahmbhatt B, Brown K, Bauce B, Muriago M, Basso C, Thiene G, Danieli GA, Rampazzo A. Identification of mutations in the cardiac ryanodine receptor gene in families affected with arrhythmogenic right ventricular cardiomyopathy type 2 (ARVD2). Hum Mol Genet 2001;10: 189–194.

136. McKoy G, Protonotarios N, Crosby A, Tsatsopoulou A, Anastasakis A, Coonar A, Norman M, Baboonian C, Jeffery S, McKenna WJ. Identification of a deletion in plakoglobin in arrhythmogenic right ventricular

cardiomyopathy with palmoplantar keratoderma and woolly hair (Naxos disease). Lancet 2000;355: 2119–2124.

137. Rampazzo A, Nava A, Malacrida S, Beffagna G, Bauce B, Rossi V, Zimbello R, Simionati B, Basso C, Thiene G, Towbin JA, Danieli GA. Mutation in human desmoplakin domain binding to plakoglobin causes a dominant form of arrhythmogenic right ventricular cardiomyopathy. Am J Hum Genet 2002;71:1200–1206.

138. McKenna WJ, Thiene G, Nava A, Fontaliran F, Blomstrom-Lundqvist C, Fontaine G, Camerini F. Diagnosis of arrhythmogenic right ventricular dysplasia/cardiomyopathy. Task Force of the Working Group Myocardial and Pericardial Disease of the European Society of Cardiology and of the Scientific Council on Cardiomyopathies of the International Society and Federation of Cardiology. Br Heart J 1994;71:215–218.

139. Marcus F, Towbin JA, Zareba W, Moss A, Calkins H, Brown M, Gear K. Arrhythmogenic right ventricular dysplasia/cardiomyopathy (ARVD/C): A multidisciplinary study: design and protocol. Circulation 2003;107:2975–2978.

140. Corrado D, Fontaine G, Marcus FI, McKenna WJ, Nava A, Thiene G, Wichter T. Arrhythmogenic right ventricular dysplasia/cardiomyopathy: Need for an international registry. Study Group on Arrhythmogenic Right Ventricular Dysplasia/Cardiomyopathy of the Working Groups on Myocardial and Pericardial Disease and Arrhythmias of the European Society of Cardiology and of the Scientific Council on Cardiomyopathies of the World Heart Federation. Circulation 2000;101:E101–E106.

141. Wichter T, Borggrefe M, Haverkamp W, Chen X, Breithardt G. Efficacy of antiarrhythmic drugs in patients with arrhythmogenic right ventricular disease: Results in patients with inducible and noninducible ventricular tachycardia. Circulation 1992;86:29–37.

142. Link MS, Wang PJ, Haugh CJ, Homoud MK, Foote CB, Costeas XB, Estes NA, III. Arrhythmogenic right ventricular dysplasia: clinical results with implantable cardioverter defibrillators. J Interv Card Electrophysiol 1997;1:41–48.

143. Tavernier R, Gevaert S, De Sutter J, De Clercq A, Rottiers H, Jordaens L, Fonteyne W. Long term results of cardioverter-defibrillator implantation in patients with right ventricular dysplasia and malignant ventricular tachyarrhythmias. Heart 2001;85:53–56.

144. Breithardt G, Wichter T, Haverkamp W, Borggrefe M, Block M, Hammel D, Scheld HH. Implantable cardioverter defibrillator therapy in patients with arrhythmogenic right ventricular cardiomyopathy, long QT syndrome, or no structural heart disease. Am Heart J 1994;127:1151–1158.

145. Corrado D, Leoni L, Link MS, Della BP, Gaita F, Curnis A, Salerno JU, Igidbashian D, Raviele A, Disertori M, Zanotto G, Verlato R, Vergara G, Delise P, Turrini P, Basso C, Naccarella F, Maddalena F, Estes NA, III, Buja G, Thiene G. Implantable cardioverter-defibrillator therapy for prevention of sudden death in patients with arrhythmogenic right ventricular cardiomyopathy/dysplasia. Circulation 2003;108:3084–91.

146. Wichter T, Paul M, Wollmann C, Acil T, Gerdes P, Ashraf O, Tjan TD, Soeparwata R, Block M, Borggrefe M, Scheld HH, Breithardt G, Böcker D. Implantable cardioverter-defibrillator therapy in arrhythmogenic

right ventricular cardiomyopathy: Single-center experience of long-term follow-up and complications in 60 patients. Circulation 2004;109:1503–8.

147. Lahat H, Eldar M, Levy-Nissenbaum E, Bahan T, Friedman E, Khoury A, Lorber A, Kastner DL, Goldman B, Pras E. Autosomal recessive catecholamine- or exercise-induced polymorphic ventricular tachycardia: Clinical features and assignment of the disease gene to chromosome 1p13-21. Circulation 2001;103:2822–2827.

148. Postma AV, Denjoy I, Hoorntje TM, Lupoglazoff JM, Da Costa A, Sebillon P, Mannens MM, Wilde AA, Guicheney P. Absence of calsequestrin 2 causes severe forms of catecholaminergic polymorphic ventricular tachycardia. Circ Res 2002;91:e21–e26.

149. Priori SG, Napolitano C, Tiso N, Memmi M, Vignati G, Bloise R, Sorrentino V, V, Danieli GA. Mutations in the cardiac ryanodine receptor gene (hRyR2) underlie catecholaminergic polymorphic ventricular tachycardia. Circulation 2001;103:196–200.

150. Marks AR, Priori S, Memmi M, Kontula K, Laitinen PJ. Involvement of the cardiac ryanodine receptor/calcium release channel in catecholaminergic polymorphic ventricular tachycardia. J Cell Physiol 2002;190:1–6.

151. Priori SG, Napolitano C, Memmi M, Colombi B, Drago F, Gasparini M, DeSimone L, Coltorti F, Bloise R, Keegan R, Cruz Filho FE, Vignati G, Benatar A, DeLogu A. Clinical and molecular characterization of patients with catecholaminergic polymorphic ventricular tachycardia. Circulation 2002;106:69–74.

152. Lahat H, Pras E, Olender T, Avidan N, Ben Asher E, Man O, Levy-Nissenbaum E, Khoury A, Lorber

A, Goldman B, Lancet D, Eldar M. A missense mutation in a highly conserved region of CASQ2 is associated with autosomal recessive catecholamine-induced polymorphic ventricular tachycardia in Bedouin families from Israel. Am J Hum Genet 2001;69:1378–1384.

153. Grimm M, Wieselthaler G, Avanessian R, Grimm G, Schmidinger H, Schreiner W, Podczeck A, Wolner E, Laufer G. The impact of implantable cardioverter-defibrillators on mortality among patients on the waiting list for heart transplantation. J Thorac Cardiovasc Surg 1995;110:532–539.

154. Sweeney MO, Ruskin JN, Garan H, McGovern BA, Guy ML, Torchiana DF, Vlahakes GJ, Newell JB, Semigran MJ, Dec GW. Influence of the implantable cardioverter/defibrillator on sudden death and total mortality in patients evaluated for cardiac transplantation. Circulation 1995;92:3273–3281.

155. Auricchio A, Stellbrink C, Sack S, Block M, Vogt J, Bakker P, Huth C, Schondube F, Wolfhard U, Böcker D, Krahnefeld O, Kirkels H. Long-term clinical effect of hemodynamically optimized cardiac resynchronization therapy in patients with heart failure and ventricular conduction delay. J Am Coll Cardiol 2002;39:2026–2033.

156. Cazeau S, Leclercq C, Lavergne T, Walker S, Varma C, Linde C, Garrigue S, Kappenberger L, Haywood GA, Santini M, Bailleul C, Daubert JC. Effects of multisite biventricular pacing in patients with heart failure and intraventricular conduction delay. N Engl J Med 2001;344:873–880.

157. Abraham WT, Fisher WG, Smith AL, DeLurgio DB, Leon AR, Loh E, Kocovic DZ, Packer M, Clavell AL, Hayes DL, Ellestad M, Trupp RJ, Underwood J,

Pickering F, Truex C, McAtee P, Messenger J. Cardiac resynchronization in chronic heart failure. N Engl J Med 2002;346:1845–1853.

158. Guerra JM, Wu J, Miller JM, Groh WJ. Increase in ventricular tachycardia frequency after biventricular implantable cardioverter defibrillator upgrade. J Cardiovasc Electrophysiol 2003;14:1245–1247.

159. Higgins SL, Yong P, Sheck D, McDaniel M, Bollinger F, Vadecha M, Desai S, Meyer DB. Biventricular pacing diminishes the need for implantable cardioverter defibrillator therapy. Ventak CHF Investigators. J Am Coll Cardiol 2000;36:824–827.

160. Walker S, Levy TM, Rex S, Brant S, Allen J, Ilsley CJ, Paul VE. Usefulness of suppression of ventricular arrhythmia by biventricular pacing in severe congestive cardiac failure. Am J Cardiol 2000;86:231–233.

161. Bradley DJ, Bradley EA, Baughman KL, Berger RD, Calkins H, Goodman SN, Kass DA, Powe NR. Cardiac resynchronization and death from progressive heart failure: a meta-analysis of randomized controlled trials. JAMA 2003;289:730–740.

162. Achilli A, Sassara M, Ficili S, Pontillo D, Achilli P, Alessi C, De Spirito S, Guerra R, Patruno N, Serra F. Long-term effectiveness of cardiac resynchronization therapy in patients with refractory heart failure and "narrow" QRS. J Am Coll Cardiol 2003;42:2117–2124.

163. Auricchio A, Stellbrink C, Butter C, Sack S, Vogt J, Misier AR, Bocker D, Block M, Kirkels JH, Kramer A, Huvelle E. Clinical efficacy of cardiac resynchronization therapy using left ventricular pacing in heart failure patients stratified by severity of

ventricular conduction delay. J Am Coll Cardiol 2003;42:2109–2116.

164. Schwartz PJ, Breithardt G, Howard AJ, Julian DG, Rehnqvist AN. Task Force Report: The legal implications of medical guidelines—A Task Force of the European Society of Cardiology. Eur Heart J 1999; 20:1152–1157.

165. Bassand JP, Ryden L. Guidelines: making the headlines or confined to the sidelines? Eur Heart J 1999; 20:1149–1151.

166. Mehta D, Saksena S, Krol RB, Makhija V. Comparison of clinical benefits and outcome in patients with programmable and nonprogrammable implantable cardioverter defibrillators. Pacing Clin Electrophysiol 1992;15:1279–1290.

167. Lehmann MH, Steinman RT, Schuger CD, Jackson K. The automatic implantable cardioverter defibrillator as antiarrhythmic treatment modality of choice for survivors of cardiac arrest unrelated to acute myocardial infarction. Am J Cardiol 1988;62:803–805.

168. Tchou PJ, Kadri N, Anderson J, Caceres JA, Jazayeri M, Akhtar M. Automatic implantable cardioverter defibrillators and survival of patients with left ventricular dysfunction and malignant ventricular arrhythmias. Ann Intern Med 1988;109:529–534.

169. Fogoros RN, Fiedler SB, Elson JJ. The automatic implantable cardioverter-defibrillator in drug- refractory ventricular tachyarrhythmias. Ann Intern Med 1987;107:635–640.

170. Powell AC, Fuchs T, Finkelstein DM, Garan H, Cannom DS, McGovern BA, Kelly E, Vlahakes GJ, Torchiana DF, Ruskin JN. Influence of implantable

cardioverter-defibrillators on the long- term prognosis of survivors of out-of-hospital cardiac arrest. Circulation 1993;88:1083–1092.

171. Crandall BG, Morris CD, Cutler JE, Kudenchuk PJ, Peterson JL, Liem LB, Broudy DR, Greene HL, Halperin BD, McAnulty JH, Kron J. Implantable cardioverter-defibrillator therapy in survivors of out-of-hospital sudden cardiac death without inducible arrhythmias. J Am Coll Cardiol 1993;21:1186–1192.

172. The PCD Investigator Group. Clinical outcome of patients with malignant ventricular tachyarrhythmias and a multiprogrammable implantable cardioverter-defibrillator implanted with or without thoracotomy: An international multicenter study. J Am Coll Cardiol 1994;23:1521–1530.

173. Zipes DP, Roberts D, Pacemaker-Cardioverter-Defibrillator Investigators. Results of the international study of the implantable pacemaker cardioverter-defibrillator. A comparison of epicardial and endocardial lead systems. Circulation 1995; 92:59–65.

174. Morady F, Harvey M, Kalbfleisch SJ, El Atassi R, Calkins H, Langberg JJ. Radiofrequency catheter ablation of ventricular tachycardia in patients with coronary artery disease. Circulation 1993;87:363–372.

175. Stevenson WG, Khan H, Sager P, Saxon LA, Middlekauff HR, Natterson PD, Wiener I. Identification of reentry circuit sites during catheter mapping and radiofrequency ablation of ventricular tachycardia late after myocardial infarction. Circulation 1993;88:1647–1670.

176. Gonska BD, Cao K, Schaumann A, Dorszewski A, von-zur MF, Kreuzer H. Catheter ablation of ventricular tachycardia in 136 patients with coronary artery

disease: results and long-term follow-up. J Am Coll Cardiol 1994;24:1506–1514.

177. Hindricks G. The Multicentre European Radiofrequency Survey (MERFS): Complications of radiofrequency catheter ablation of arrhythmias. Eur Heart J 1993;14:1644–1653.

178. Bardy GH, Yee R, Jung W, Active Can Investigators. Multicenter experience with a pectoral unipolar implantable cardioverter-defibrillator. Active Can Investigators. J Am Coll Cardiol 1996;28:400–410.

179. Groh WJ, Silka MJ, Oliver RP, Halperin BD, McAnulty JH, Kron J. Use of implantable cardioverter-defibrillators in the congenital long QT syndrome. Am J Cardiol 1996;78:703–706.

180. Michaud GF, Sticherling C, Tada H, Oral H, Pelosi F, Jr., Knight BP, Morady F, Strickberger SA. Relationship between serum potassium concentration and risk of recurrent ventricular tachycardia or ventricular fibrillation. J Cardiovasc Electrophysiol 2001;12:1109–1112.

181. Michaud GF, Strickberger SA. Should an abnormal serum potassium concentration be considered a correctable cause of cardiac arrest? J Am Coll Cardiol 2001;38:1224–1225.

182. Saksena S, Breithardt G, Dorian P, Greene HL, Madan N, Block M. Nonpharmacological therapy for malignant ventricular arrhythmias: implantable defibrillator trials. Prog Cardiovasc Dis 1996;38:429–444.

183. Brugada J, Brugada R, Brugada P. Pharmacological and device approach to therapy of inherited cardiac diseases associated with cardiac arrhythmias and sudden death. J Electrocardiol 2000;33 (Suppl):41–47.

184. Vlay SC, Olson LC, Fricchione GL, Friedman R. Anxiety and anger in patients with ventricular tachyarrhythmias. Responses after automatic internal cardioverter defibrillator implantation. Pacing Clin Electrophysiol 1989;12:366–373.
185. Lüderitz B, Jung W, Deister A, Marneros A, Manz M. Patient acceptance of the implantable cardioverter defibrillator in ventricular tachyarrhythmias. Pacing Clin Electrophysiol 1993;16:1815–1821.

Index

Page numbers in *italics* represent figures, those in **bold** represent tables.